FOURTH EDITION

THE
ECG
IN PRACTICE

Commissioning Editor: Laurence Hunter
Project Development Manager: Lynn Watt and Helius
Project Manager: Nancy Arnott
Designer: Erik Bigland and Helius
Illustrator: Gecko Ltd and Helius
Illustration Manager: Bruce Hogarth

FOURTH EDITION

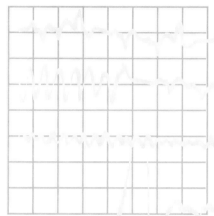

THE

ECG
IN PRACTICE

John R. Hampton DM MA DPhil FRCP FFPM FESC

Emeritus Professor of Cardiology
University of Nottingham
Nottingham
UK

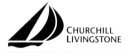
CHURCHILL
LIVINGSTONE

EDINBURGH LONDON NEW YORK OXFORD PHILADELPHIA
ST LOUIS SYDNEY TORONTO 2003

CHURCHILL LIVINGSTONE An imprint of Elsevier Science Limited

© Longman Education UK Limited 1986, 1992
© Pearson Professional Limited 1997
© 2003, Elsevier Science Limited. All rights reserved.

First edition 1986
Second edition 1992
Third edition 1997
Fourth edition 2003
   Reprinted 2003

Standard edition ISBN 0 443 072507
International edition ISBN 0 443 072515

British Library Cataloguing in Publication Data
A catalogue record for this book is available from the British Library

Library of Congress Cataloging in Publication Data
A catalog record for this book is available from the Library of Congress

Note
Medical knowledge is constantly changing. Standard safety precautions must be followed, but as new research and clinical experience broaden our knowledge, changes in treatment and drug therapy may become necessary or appropriate. Readers are advised to check the most current product information provided by the manufacturer of each drug to be administered to verify the recommended dose, the method and duration of administration, and contraindications. It is the responsibility of the practitioner, relying on experience and knowledge of the patient, to determine dosages and the best treatment for each individual patient. Neither the Publisher nor the author assumes any liability for any injury and/or damage to persons or property arising from this publication.

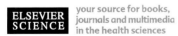

ELSEVIER SCIENCE your source for books, journals and multimedia in the health sciences

www.elsevierhealth.com

The publisher's policy is to use paper manufactured from sustainable forests

Printed in China
P/02

Preface

What to expect of this book

I assume that the reader of this book will have the level of
knowledge of the ECG that is contained in *The ECG Made Easy*, to
which this is a companion volume. The ECG is indeed easy in
principle, but the variations in pattern seen both in normal people
and in patients with cardiac and other problems can make the
ECG seem more complex than it really is. This book concentrates
on these variations, and contains several examples of each
abnormality. It is thus intended for anyone who understands the
basics, but now wants to use the ECG to its maximum potential as
a clinical tool.

The ECG is not an end in itself, but is an extension of the history
and physical examination. Patients do not visit the doctor wanting
an ECG, but come either for a health check or because they have
symptoms. Therefore this book is organized according to clinical
situations, and the chapters cover the ECG in healthy subjects and
in patients with palpitations, syncope, chest pain, breathlessness
or non-cardiac diseases. To emphasize that the ECG is part of the
general assessment of a patient, each chapter begins with a brief
section on history and examination and ends with a short account
of what might be done once the ECG has been interpreted.

This edition adopts the philosophy of its predecessors regarding
the relative importance of the ECG and the individual in whom it
was recorded, but most of the illustrations are new and there is
now an emphasis on 12-lead ECGs, reproduced as realistically as is
possible in a small book. It begins with revision of *The ECG Made
Easy*, extended to cover the physiology and pathophysiology
underlying ECG patterns.

What to expect of the ECG

The ECG has its limitations. Remember that it provides a picture
of the electrical activity of the heart, but gives only an indirect
indication of the heart's structure and function. It is, however,
invaluable for assessing patients whose symptoms may be due to

electrical malfunction, including patients with conduction problems and those with arrhythmias.

In healthy people, finding the ECG to be normal may be reassuring. Unfortunately the ECG can be totally normal in patients with severe coronary disease. Conversely, the range of normality is such that a healthy subject may quite wrongly be labelled as having heart disease on the basis of the ECG. Some ECG patterns that are undoubtedly abnormal (for example, right bundle branch block) are seen in perfectly healthy people. It is a good working principle that it is the individual's clinical state that matters, not the ECG.

When a patient complains of palpitations or syncope, the diagnosis of a cardiac cause is only certain if an ECG is recorded at the time of symptoms – but even when the patient is symptom-free, the ECG may provide a clue for the prepared mind. In patients with chest pain the ECG may make the diagnosis and treatment can be based upon it, but it is essential to remember that the ECG may remain normal for a few hours after the onset of a myocardial infarction. In breathless patients a totally normal ECG probably rules out heart failure, but it is not a good way of diagnosing lung disease or pulmonary embolism. Finally it must be remembered that the ECG can be quite abnormal in a patient with a variety of non-cardiac diseases, and one must not jump to the conclusion that an abnormal ECG indicates cardiac pathology.

How to report an ECG

The ECG is most valuable when the reasons for it being recorded are known – as always in medicine, it is better to look *for* things than *at* things. An ECG report should have two parts: a description, which is a matter of fact, and an interpretation. The description should include the rhythm, the rate, the axis and an account of the QRS complexes, ST segments and T waves. The interpretation should include a list of possible reasons for any abnormalities described. Try to look at all the ECGs in this book and report them to yourself in this way.

Acknowledgements

I have tried to include examples of most of the normal ECG variations, and of most of the abnormalities, that will be encountered in day-to-day practice. I am extremely grateful to many friends and colleagues who have helped me to find them.

John R. Hampton
Nottingham

Contents

General contents

Medical conditions illustrated by 12-lead ECGs

1

Revision course: the ECG is easy

ANATOMY AND PHYSIOLOGY

The anatomy underlying the ECG is easy (Fig. 1.1).

Excitation, or depolarization, usually begins in the sinoatrial (SA) node. It spreads as a wave through the atrial muscle, but cannot directly penetrate the ventricular muscle because the atria are 'insulated' from the ventricle. The only normal connection between the two is via the atrioventricular node (the AV node, or simply 'the node'), the His bundle and its branches, and the Purkinje fibres. These different structures conduct depolarization at different speeds:

1

- atrial muscle: 1 metre per second (m/s)
- AV node: 0.2 m/s
- His bundle, bundle branches and Purkinje tissue: 4.0 m/s
- ventricular muscle: 0.5 m/s.

The P wave of the ECG represents depolarization (remember: depolarization, not contraction) of the atria. The PR interval represents conduction through the AV node and the His bundle, and measures the time taken for the depolarization wave to spread from the atria to the interventricular septum, which is the first part of the ventricles to depolarize. The QRS complex represents depolarization of the ventricles, and the T wave represents ventricular muscle repolarization (Fig. 1.2).

Normally each heartbeat involves one P wave per QRS complex and a QRS complex can have only one associated T wave. If there are more P waves than QRS complexes, there must be a disorder of conduction.

The time taken by each of these sections of the ECG complex can be measured from the ECG paper. At the normal paper speed of 25 mm/s, one large square represents 200 ms and one small square represents 40 ms. The normal limits are:

- PR interval: 120–200 ms (less than 120 ms suggests an abnormal connection between atria and ventricles or 'pre-excitation', and more than 200 ms indicates a conduction 'block')
- QRS complex: less than 120 ms (more means a slow spread of depolarization through the ventricular muscle)

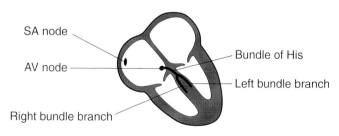

SA node
AV node
Bundle of His
Left bundle branch
Right bundle branch

Fig. 1.1 The wiring diagram of the heart

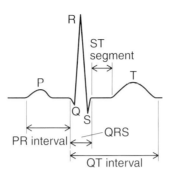

Fig. 1.2 The components of the ECG complex

- T wave: duration is difficult to measure and the QT interval is usually taken as the best indication of the time taken for repolarization of the ventricles. The height of the T wave and the QT interval are affected by many things, including the direction of spread of the preceding depolarization, ischaemia, infarction and electrolyte disturbance. These variations in the T wave have to be learned rather than deduced.

THE 12-LEAD ECG

The 12 'leads' that make up the standard ECG 'look at' the heart from different directions. Each cycle of depolarization looks different in each of the 12 leads because:

- depolarization spreading towards a lead causes an upward deflection
- depolarization spreading away from a lead causes a downward deflection.

The limb leads 'look at' the heart in a vertical plane from the sides, above and below. Seen from the front, the average deflection of the depolarization waves in the ventricle spreads from 10 o'clock to 4 o'clock. It is therefore moving away from VR and towards VL, I, II and III. This is called the cardiac axis, and in

3

the normal heart the QRS complex is predominantly downward in VR (that is, the S wave exceeds the R wave) but predominantly upward in the other limb leads (the R wave is bigger than any S wave that may be present). Thus when the axis is normal, the QRS complex is predominantly upright in leads I, II and III (Fig. 1.3).

If the axis swings to the right the QRS complex becomes predominantly downward in lead I but remains predominantly upward in leads II and III. If the axis swings to the left, the QRS complex is upright in lead I but downward in leads II and III.

The chest leads 'look at' the heart in a horizontal plane from the front and the left side. Leads V_1 and V_2 overlie and therefore 'look at' the right ventricle, V_3 and V_4 are over the interventricular septum, and V_5 and V_6 are over the left ventricle. Because the left ventricle is more muscular than the right, it has more effect on the ECG. Lead V_1 therefore 'sees' the difference between depolarization spreading towards it in the right ventricle and

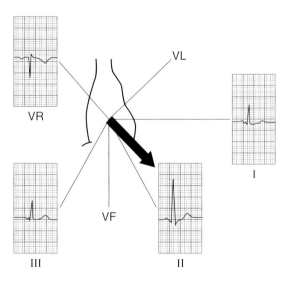

Fig. 1.3 Normal axis

away from it in the left ventricle. The net result is a spread of depolarization away from V_1, and V_1 therefore records a predominantly downward deflection. Lead V_6 'sees' the main depolarization of the left ventricle spreading towards it, with the smaller depolarization due to the right ventricle spreading away from it, so the result is an upright QRS complex (Fig. 1.4). If the heart is swung round so that the right ventricle occupies more of

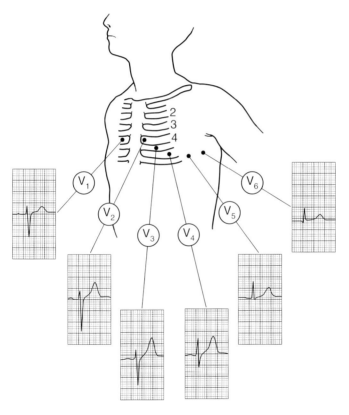

Fig. 1.4 The chest leads. Note that the rib spaces are numbered

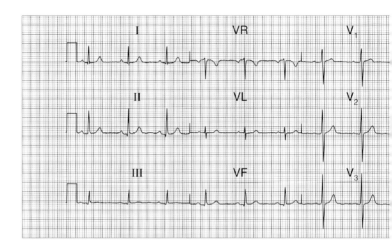

the front of the chest than usual, it may be necessary to position the chest leads in the axilla and on the back (leads V_7, V_8 and V_9) to obtain a 'left ventricular complex' in the ECG. This is called 'clockwise rotation', and is common in chronic lung disease.

Figure 1.5 shows a normal 12-lead ECG. Look at the appearance of the P, QRS and T waves in each lead. Remember that they each show a different 'view' of a cycle of depolarization and repolarization. You will have to become very familiar with this pattern.

REPORTING AN ECG

An ECG report has two parts: a description and an interpretation. The description must include:

- where depolarization started – the 'rhythm'. Normally this will be sinoatrial, i.e. 'sinus rhythm'
- whether conduction of depolarization occurred normally
- whether the axis is normal, left, or right
- an account of the QRS complex shape and duration
- description of the T wave in the different leads.

In Figure 1.5 the description is thus:

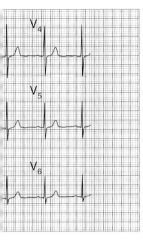

Fig. 1.5 The normal ECG

- sinus rhythm
- normal axis
- normal conduction
- normal QRS complexes
- normal T waves.

The interpretation is: normal record.

CONDUCTION DEFECTS

In this section we will assume that depolarization begins in the SA node, so the heart is in sinus rhythm. Any lead can be used to show the cardiac rhythm on the ECG. In practice, the rhythm is determined from the lead that shows the P wave most clearly.

The conduction of depolarization can be delayed or 'blocked' anywhere along the pathway from the SA node to the ventricular muscle, and the sites of conduction defects can usually be deduced from the surface ECG (Fig. 1.6).

Sinoatrial block

In sinoatrial block, the SA node depolarizes normally but the depolarization wave fails to penetrate the atrium (Fig. 1.7).

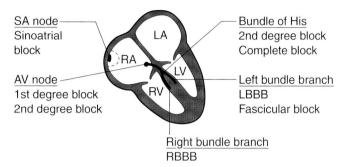

Fig. 1.6 Possible sites for conduction block

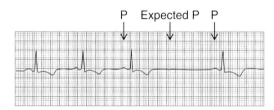

Fig. 1.7 Sinoatrial block

Note
- Sinus rhythm for three beats, then a 'sinus pause'
- P waves arrowed
- The expected P wave is not seen, but the SA node must have been depolarized because the next P wave appears at the predicted time

Intra-atrial conduction delay

Depolarization spreads throughout the atrial muscle, so conduction defects do not occur there. However, activation of the whole of the atrial myocardium may take longer than normal if the left atrium is hypertrophied. This causes the broad bifid P wave seen in the ECGs of patients with mitral stenosis, as long as they remain in sinus rhythm (Ch.5).

Atrioventricular node and His bundle block

The PR interval (the period from the onset of the P wave to the first deflection of the QRS complex) measures the time taken for the depolarization wave to spread from the SA node, through the atria and the AV node, and down the His bundle to the interventricular septum. If the PR interval is prolonged, or if the P wave is not followed by a QRS complex, a conduction defect must be present either in the AV node itself or in the His bundle. It is not possible to tell from the surface ECG which of these two sites is involved.

The passage of the depolarization wave down the His bundle can be detected if an electrode is placed close to the His bundle: this can be done by passing an electrode catheter up a femoral vein and positioning it just through the tricuspid valve. The electrical activity associated with atrial depolarization recorded in this way is called an 'A' wave rather than a P wave, and that associated with ventricular depolarization is called a 'V' wave rather than a QRS complex (Fig. 1.8). Depolarization of the His bundle itself is shown as a sharp deflection called the 'H spike'.

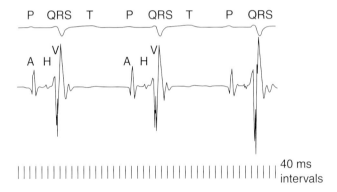

Fig. 1.8 Normal His bundle electrogram

Note
- Upper trace shows the usual ECG recorded from the body surface
- The P waves, QRS complexes and T waves are broad and flat because the record was made with a fast paper speed
- The lower trace shows the intracardiac recording. The A and V waves correspond to the P waves and QRS complexes, but have a totally different appearance
- His bundle depolarization is shown as a small spike labelled 'H'

The AH interval thus measures the time taken for the depolarization wave to spread from the SA node to the His bundle. Most of this period is due to delay within the AV node. In normal subjects the AH interval is between 55 and 120 ms. The HV interval (normal range 35–55 ms) measures the time taken for depolarization to spread from the His bundle to the first part of the interventricular septum.

First degree block

When each atrial depolarization is followed by ventricular depolarization but atrioventricular conduction is slow, the PR interval on the surface ECG is prolonged and 'first degree block' is said to be present (Fig. 1.9). This can be seen in normal people but may indicate many varieties of heart disease (e.g. acute myocardial infarction, acute rheumatic carditis). However, in itself it does not impair cardiac function, and does not cause symptoms.

First degree block commonly occurs in the AV node. A His bundle electrogram therefore records a prolonged AH interval but a normal HV interval, because conduction in the distal part of the His bundle is normal (Fig. 1.10).

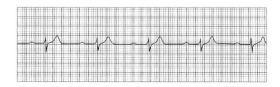

Fig. 1.9 First degree block

Note
- Sinus rhythm
- PR interval is constant (360 ms)

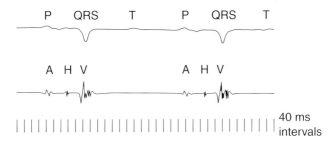

Fig. 1.10 His electrogram: first degree block

Note
- Upper record shows surface ECG
- The PR interval is 200 ms
- Lower record shows His electrogram
- The AH interval is prolonged (150 ms), but the HV interval is normal (70 ms)

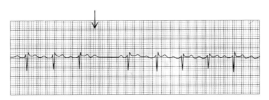

Fig. 1.11 Second degree block (Mobitz type 2)

Note
- Sinus rhythm with a normal PR interval
- One P wave (arrowed) is not followed by a QRS complex

Second degree block

When atrial depolarization intermittently fails to induce ventricular depolarization, 'second degree block' exists. This can result from conduction failure anywhere in the AV node or His bundle. There are three varieties:

1. When most beats are conducted normally but occasionally a P wave is not followed by a QRS complex, second degree block of the 'Mobitz type 2' variety is said to be present (Fig. 1.11). The

11

conduction defect is thought to be below the AV node, in the bundle of His. This does not in itself cause symptoms, and its only importance is that it may precede the development of complete block.

2. When the PR interval lengthens progressively with each beat and then a P wave is not conducted and so is not followed by a QRS complex, the 'Wenckebach phenomenon' is present (Fig. 1.12). The conduction abnormality in this case is within the AV node.

3. When alternate P waves are not conducted, second degree block of the '2:1' type is said to be present (Fig. 1.13).

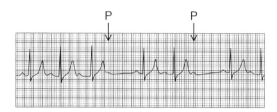

Fig. 1.12 Second degree block (Wenckebach)

Note
- Three beats with progressively longer PR intervals are followed by a non-conducted P wave (arrowed)
- The next PR interval is short, but this is followed by a longer PR interval and then another non-conducted beat

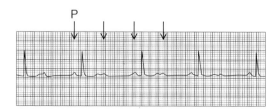

Fig. 1.13 Second degree block (2:1)

Note
- The conducted beats have a normal PR interval
- Alternate P waves are not followed by a QRS complex

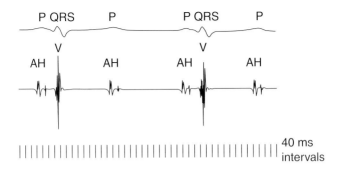

Fig. 1.14 His electrogram: second degree block

Note
- Upper trace shows the surface ECG
- As in the case of the other His electrograms the paper speed is fast, so the P–QRS–T complexes are flattened and spread out
- Lower trace shows first a normal A wave, H spike and V wave, but then an A wave and an H spike with no V wave
- The sequence is then repeated

The His bundle electrogram demonstrates the site of second degree block. In the case of 2:1 block this is usually in the His bundle rather than the AV node – so a normal H (or His) spike will be seen, but in the non-conducted beats the H spike will not be followed by a V wave (Fig. 1.14).

Second degree blocks of the Mobitz 2 and Wenckebach types do not cause symptoms, but 2:1 block may cause heart failure if the ventricular rate is slow enough.

Third degree block
Third degree, or complete, heart block results either from His bundle disease or from bilateral bundle branch block. A narrow QRS complex indicates that the rhythm originates within the His bundle itself below the block, but a wide QRS complex indicates that ventricular depolarization originates in the Purkinje system (Fig. 1.15).

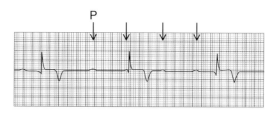

Fig. 1.15 Complete (third degree) block

Note

- No relationship between P waves (arrowed) and QRS complexes
- The QRS complexes are normal, indicating that the origin of ventricular depolarization is within the His bundle
- The ventricular rate is 30/min

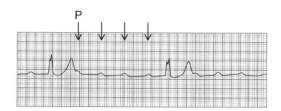

Fig 1.16 Complete (third Degree) block

Note

- No relationship between P waves (arrowed) and QRS complexes
- Wide QRS complexes
- Ventricular rate of 22/min

When complete heart block complicates an acute inferior infarction, the ventricular rate is usually about 50/min. The classical ventricular escape rate of 20–30/min is usually seen when complete block results from fibrosis of the His bundle (Fig. 1.16).

Complete heart block does impair cardiac performance: the effect of synchronized atrial and ventricular contraction is lost and, more importantly, cardiac output falls because of the slow heart rate.

Bundle branch block

When the His bundle conducts normally but one of the bundle branches is blocked, the PR interval is normal but the QRS complex is widened because of the late depolarization of the part of the ventricle normally supplied by the bundle branch which is blocked. Bundle branch block does not significantly impair cardiac function, and in itself will not be responsible for any symptoms the patient may have.

Right bundle branch block (RBBB) is characterized by an RSR[1] pattern in lead V_1 (Fig. 1.17). An R[1] is a secondary R wave: a first upward deflection is an R, but a secondary upward deflection after an S wave is called an R[1].

Left bundle branch block (LBBB) is characterized by a loss of the septal Q wave (see Ch. 2) and the notching of the QRS complex in the lateral leads (Fig. 1.18).

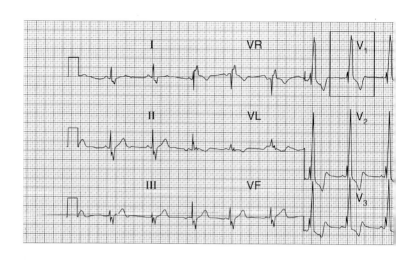

Fig. 1.18 Left bundle branch block

Note

- Sinus rhythm
- Broad QRS complexes with notch in the R wave in I, VL, V₅, V₆
- Inverted T waves are associated with bundle branch block, and have no other significance

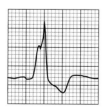

Notched R wave in lead V₆

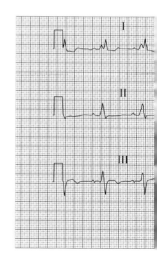

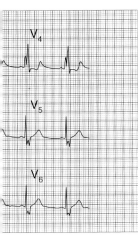

Fig. 1.17 Right bundle branch block

Note
- Sinus rhythm with a normal PR interval
- RSR^1 pattern in V$_1$
- The dominant R wave is characteristic of RBBB, and does not indicate RV hypertrophy
- Wide and slurred S wave in V$_6$

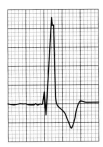

RSR^1 pattern in lead V$_1$

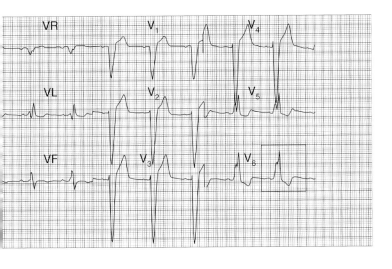

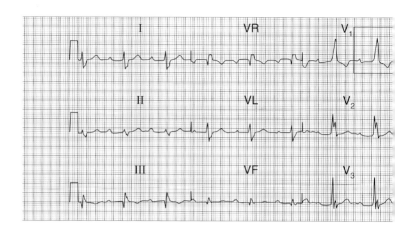

If a bundle branch block is associated with first degree block, it is likely that either the His bundle or the remaining bundle branch is diseased and that bilateral bundle branch block (causing third degree block) may develop. Figure 1.19 shows first degree block and RBBB.

Fascicular block

The right bundle branch is a single structure, but the left bundle branch divides into two further branches or fascicles. Depolarization spreads into the left ventricle through these fascicles, and the average of these two directions of depolarization as seen from the front is called the frontal plane vector or cardiac axis (Fig. 1.20).

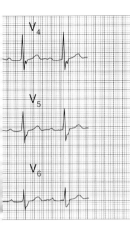

Fig. 1.19 First degree block and right bundle branch block

Note
- Sinus rhythm
- PR interval 320 ms (first degree block)
- Broad QRS complexes
- RSR^1 pattern best seen in V$_2$
- Wide slurred S in V$_6$

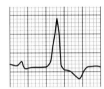

Long PR interval and broad QRS complex with dominant R wave in lead V$_1$

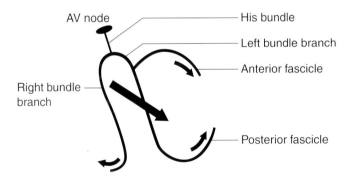

Fig. 1.20 The normal cardiac axis

Note
- Small arrows show the direction of spread of depolarization through the main branches of the His bundle
- Broad arrow shows the average direction of spread of depolarization in these three branches as seen from the front
- This average direction is the cardiac axis

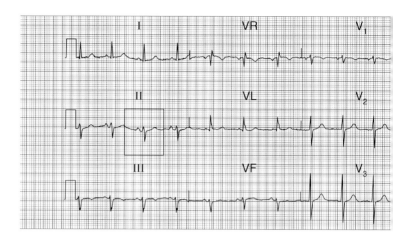

Failure of conduction in the antero-superior branch of the left bundle (left anterior fascicular block or 'left anterior hemiblock') means that the left ventricle has to be depolarized through the posterior fascicle. The average direction of depolarization, the cardiac axis, therefore swings upward and causes left axis deviation (Fig. 1.21).

Failure of conduction in the posterior inferior fascicle (left posterior hemiblock) causes the cardiac axis to swing to the right, and this is shown by a deep S wave in lead I. This is seen much less often than left anterior hemiblock. Left posterior hemiblock can be recognized by the association of right axis deviation and some evidence of left ventricular disease, without anything to suggest right ventricular hypertrophy.

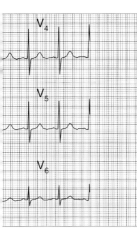

Fig. 1.21 Left anterior hemiblock

Note
- Sinus rhythm with a normal PR interval
- Average direction of depolarization in the standard leads is towards I, and away from both II and III
- Leads II and III show dominant S waves

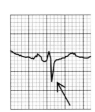

Deep S wave wave in lead II

Bifascicular block

A combination of RBBB and left anterior hemiblock indicates disease of two of the three main ventricular conduction pathways. This is an example of 'bifascicular' block (Fig. 1.22).

Trifascicular block

If all three fascicles completely fail to conduct, the effect is the same as complete failure of the His bundle – complete or third degree block. It is only possible to tell whether it is His bundle block or three-fascicle block by intracardiac recording.

However when bifascicular block is established, delayed conduction in the remaining fascicle (or in the His bundle) may cause first degree block. The combination of first degree block and bifascicular block is sometimes called (perhaps inaccurately) trifascicular block (Fig. 1.23).

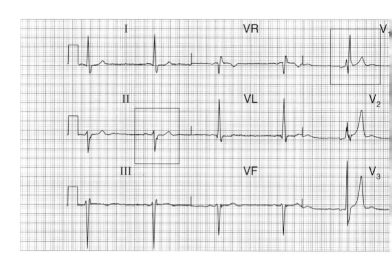

Fig. 1.23 Trifascicular block

Note
- PR interval 280 ms
- Left axis deviation
- Broad QRS complexes
- RSR^1 pattern in V$_1$

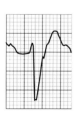

Left axis deviation, left anterior hemiblock and first degree block wave in lead II

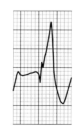

RBBB and first degree block wave in lead V$_1$

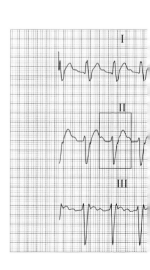

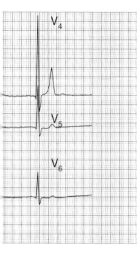

Fig. 1.22 Bifascicular block

Note

- Sinus rhythm with a normal PR interval
- Left axis deviation
- RSR[1] pattern in V_1 and a wide S wave in V_6 indicate RBBB

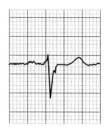

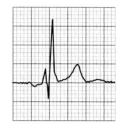

Left axis deviation wave in lead II

RBBB wave in lead V_1

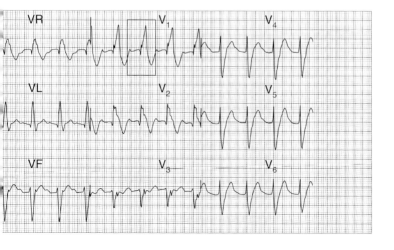

THE CARDIAC RHYTHM

The word 'rhythm' describes the part of the heart that initiates, and therefore controls, the spread of depolarization. In the normal heart depolarization begins in the SA node and the rhythm is 'sinus rhythm'. If depolarization begins in the atria or the AV node we have 'atrial' or 'AV nodal' (often called 'junctional') rhythm. Depolarization beginning in the ventricles causes 'ventricular' rhythm. Any rhythm other than sinus rhythm is called an 'arrhythmia'. The term 'dysrhythmia' – which means essentially the same thing – has been dropped. Properly speaking, conduction disorders are not arrhythmias.

Disorders of the sinoatrial node

'Sinus arrhythmia' is really a contradiction in terms because sinus rhythm is not an arrhythmia. The frequency of depolarization of the SA node is affected by the vagus nerve, and inspiration and expiration cause its rate of discharge to increase and decrease respectively. The normal heart is thus a little irregular – hence 'arrhythmia' (Fig. 1.24). This vagal effect diminishes with increasing age and is lost in autonomic neuropathy.

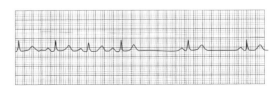

Fig. 1.24 Sinus arrhythmia

Note
- Although the R–R interval varies markedly, the shape of the P waves and the duration of the PR intervals are constant
- The irregularity in the rate of the QRS complexes must therefore be due to sinus arrhythmia

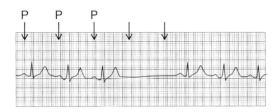

Fig. 1.25 Sinus arrest

Note
- Sinus rhythm
- After three beats there is a 'sinus pause' with no P wave
- Arrows mark where the next two P waves should have been
- Sinus rhythm is then restored, but the cycle has been reset

Loss of SA node activity causes 'sinus arrest', a rhythm common in the sick sinus syndrome (see Ch. 3). This ECG abnormality can be differentiated from SA block (the other cause of a 'sinus pause') because from time to time the expected P wave does not appear until after two (or three) normal intervals, and then not at the expected time (Fig. 1.25).

Supraventricular and ventricular rhythms

Rhythms can be grouped into those that begin 'above' the ventricles – in the SA node, atrial muscle or AV node – and are called 'supraventricular', and those that begin in the ventricular muscle and are called 'ventricular' (Figs 1.26 and 1.27). This grouping is useful because it makes identification of the arrhythmia easier, and so helps guide treatment.

In supraventricular rhythms depolarization spreads normally into the ventricles, whether it has begun in the SA node, the atrial muscle or the AV node. The QRS complex is thus the same in each of these rhythms: it is narrow and normally shaped. Ventricular repolarization is normal, so the T wave is a normal shape. In ventricular rhythms depolarization spreads relatively slowly through the ventricular muscle, so the QRS complex is wide and abnormal. Repolarization is also abnormal, so the T wave is often inverted.

25

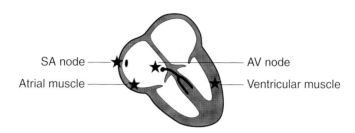

Fig. 1.26 Origins of cardiac rhythm

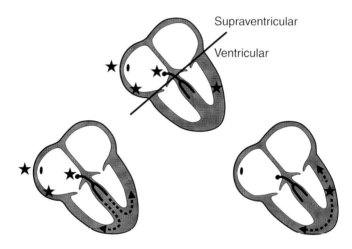

Fig. 1.27 Supraventricular and ventricular rhythms

Arrhythmias can be of the following types:

• single early beats – extrasystoles (also called premature contractions or 'ectopics'), which can be supraventricular or ventricular
• single late beats (supraventricular or ventricular – 'escape' beats)
• sustained tachycardias (again, supraventricular or ventricular)
• sustained escape rhythm.

Extrasystoles and tachycardias

Figures 1.28, 1.29 and 1.30 show examples of supraventricular extrasystoles and a supraventricular (in this case AV nodal) tachycardia. In all of these the QRS complex is narrow and the T waves are normal.

After conversion to sinus rhythm, the QRS complexes and T waves remain unchanged (Fig. 1.31).

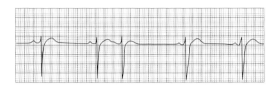

Fig. 1.28 Atrial extrasystole

Note
• Abnormally-shaped P wave

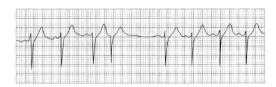

Fig. 1.29 Junctional (AV nodal) extrasystole

Note
• Usually shows no P wave

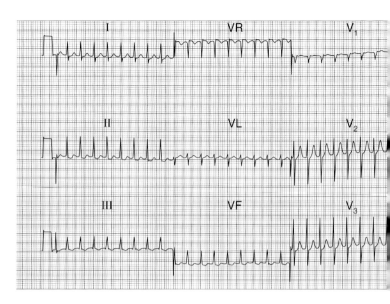

Fig. 1.31 Sinus rhythm

Note
- Same patient as in Figure 1.30
- QRS complexes and T waves unchanged

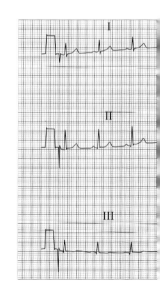

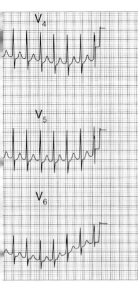

Fig. 1.30 Supraventricular tachycardia

Note
- Narrow complex tachycardia, rate 190/min
- No P waves
- Some ST segment depression, but upright T waves

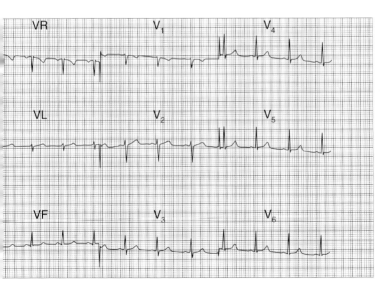

Figures 1.32 and 1.33 show ventricular extrasystoles and ventricular tachycardia respectively, and in these rhythms the QRS complexes are wide.

It is important to differentiate between beats of ventricular origin and beats that are supraventricular but show a wide QRS complex due to bundle branch block. The presence of a P wave is usually the clue.

Bundle branch block can be rate-dependent: in some patients it can occur at a high sinus rate but not at a low rate. Figure 1.34 shows sinus rhythm with wide and abnormal complexes, changing to quite different narrow complexes as the rate slows and conduction into the ventricles occurs normally.

Fig. 1.33 Ventricular tachycardia

Note
- Recording at half sensitivity
- No P waves visible
- Wide and abnormal QRS complexes
- Rate about 200/min
- T waves cannot be distinguished

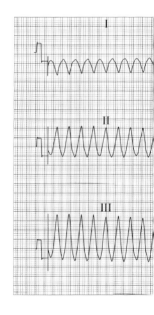

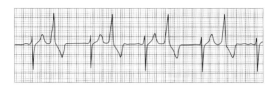

Fig. 1.32 Ventricular extrasystoles

Note
- Each sinus beat is followed by a beat with no P wave, a wide QRS complex and an inverted T wave
- This is sometimes called 'bigeminy'

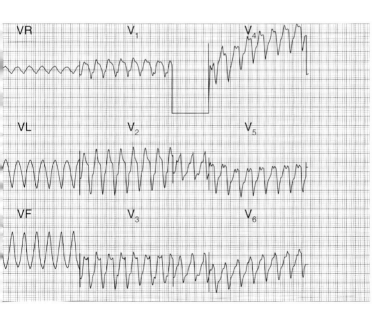

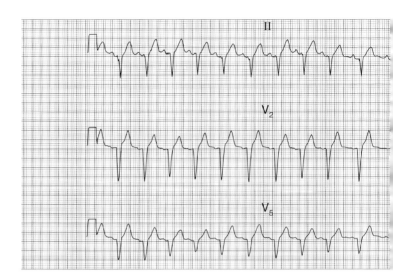

RHYTHMS RESULTING FROM CARDIAC AUTOMATICITY

Myocardial cells are only depolarized when they are stimulated, but the cells of the SA node, those around the AV node (the 'junctional' cells) and those of the conducting pathways all possess the property of spontaneous depolarization or 'automaticity'.

Escape beats

The automaticity of any part of the heart is suppressed by the arrival of a depolarization wave, and so the heart rate is controlled by the region with the highest automatic depolarization frequency. Normally the SA node controls the heart rate because it has the highest frequency of discharge but if for any reason this fails, the region with the next highest intrinsic depolarization frequency will emerge as the pacemaker and set up an 'escape' rhythm. The atria and the junctional region have automatic depolarization frequencies of about 50/min, compared with the normal SA node frequency of 60–70/min. If both the SA node and the junctional region fail to depolarize, or if conduction to the ventricles fails, a

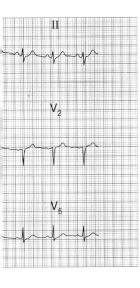

Fig. 1.34 Rate-dependent bundle branch block

Note
- Three-lead trace
- Sinus rhythm throughout
- The first ten complexes are wide: bundle branch block, not clear if right or left
- QRS complexes then become narrow as the rate slows
- This is 'rate-dependent bundle branch block'

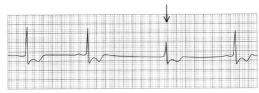

Fig. 1.35 Junctional escape beat

Note
- After two sinus beats there is no P wave
- After an interval there is a narrow QRS complex, with the same configuration as that of the sinus beats but without a preceding P wave
- This is a junctional beat (arrowed)
- Sinus rhythm then reappears

ventricular focus may emerge, with a rate of 30–40/min; this is classically seen in complete heart block.

Escape beats may be single or may form sustained rhythms. They have the same ECG appearance as the corresponding extrasystoles, but appear late rather than early (Fig. 1.35).

In sustained junctional escape rhythms, atrial activation may be seen as a P wave following the QRS complex (Fig. 1.36). This occurs if depolarization spreads in the opposite direction from normal, from the AV node to the atria, and is called 'retrograde' conduction. Figure 1.37 also shows a junctional escape rhythm.

Figure 1.38 shows a ventricular escape beat.

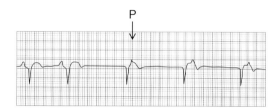

Fig. 1.36 Junctional (escape) rhythm

Note
- Two sinus beats are followed by an interval with no P waves
- A junctional rhythm then emerges (with QRS complexes the same as in sinus rhythm)
- A P wave (arrowed) can be seen as a hump on the T wave of the junctional beats: the atria have been depolarized retrogradely

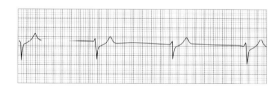

Fig. 1.37 Junctional (escape) rhythm

Note
- No P waves
- Narrow QRS complexes and normal T waves

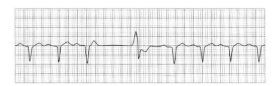

Fig. 1.38 Ventricular escape beat

Note
- Three sinus beats are followed by a pause
- There is then a single ventricular beat with a wide QRS complex and an inverted T wave
- Sinus rhythm is then restored

CAUSES OF ARRHYTHMIAS

Arrhythmias occur either because of an abnormality in the intrinsic automaticity of the heart, or because re-entry circuits are set up.

Enhanced automaticity
If the intrinsic frequency of depolarization of the atrial, junctional or ventricular conducting tissue is increased, an abnormal rhythm may occur: this phenomenon is called 'enhanced automaticity'. Single early beats, or extrasystoles, may be due to enhanced automaticity. The most common example of a sustained rhythm due to enhanced automaticity is 'accelerated idioventricular rhythm', which is common after acute myocardial infarction. The ECG appearance (Fig. 1.39) resembles that of a slow ventricular tachycardia, and that is the old-fashioned name for this condition. This rhythm causes no symptoms, and should not be treated.

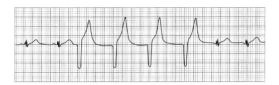

Fig. 1.39 Accelerated idioventricular rhythm

Note
- After two sinus beats, there are four beats of ventricular origin with a rate of 75/min
- Sinus rhythm is then restored

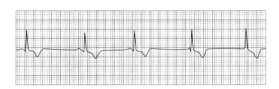

Fig. 1.40 Accelerated idionodal rhythm

Note
- After three sinus beats the sinus rate slows slightly
- A nodal rhythm appears and 'overtakes' the P waves

If the junctional intrinsic frequency is enhanced to a point at which it approximates to that of the SA node, an accelerated idionodal rhythm results. This may appear to 'overtake' the P waves (Fig. 1.40). This rhythm used to be called a 'wandering pacemaker'.

Enhanced automaticity is thought to be the mechanism causing some non-paroxysmal tachycardias, particularly those due to digoxin intoxication.

Abnormalities of cardiac rhythm due to re-entry

Normal conduction results in the uniform spread of the depolarization wave front in a constant direction. Should the direction of depolarization be reversed in some part of the heart, it becomes possible for a circular or 're-entry' pathway to be set up (Fig. 1.41). Depolarization reverberates round the pathway, causing a tachycardia. The anatomical requirement for this is the branching and rejoining of a conduction pathway. Normally, conduction is anterograde (forward) in both limbs of such a pathway, but an anterograde impulse may pass normally down one branch and be blocked in the other. From the point at which the pathways rejoin, the depolarization wave can spread retrogradely (backwards) up the abnormal branch. If it arrives when that pathway is not refractory to conduction, it can then pass right around the circuit and reactivate it.

Once established, a circular wave of depolarization may continue until some part of the pathway fails to conduct. The conduction of a depolarization wave round a circular pathway may also be interrupted by the arrival of another depolarization wave, set up by an ectopic focus (i.e. an extrasystole).

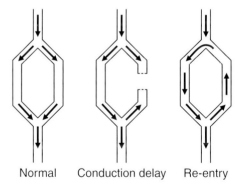

Normal   Conduction delay   Re-entry

Fig. 1.41 Re-entry mechanism causing tachycardia

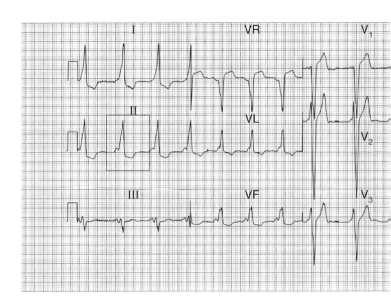

Atrioventricular re-entry (AVRE) tachycardia
The classical, though not the most common, example of re-entry
occurs in the Wolff–Parkinson–White (WPW) syndrome. Here
there is an extra, or 'accessory' conducting pathway which
connects either the right atrium to the right ventricle, or the left
atrium to the left ventricle, bypassing the AV node. The normal
delay to conduction imposed by the AV node is therefore lost,
ventricular depolarization occurs early and the PR interval is short.
Early ventricular depolarization causes a slurred upstroke to the
QRS complex, and this slurring is called a delta wave (Fig. 1.42).

The re-entry circuit comprises the normal AV node–His bundle
connection between the atria and the ventricles, and the accessory
pathway. Depolarization can spread down the normal pathway
and back (i.e. retrogradely) up through the accessory pathway to
reactivate the atria and so cause a tachycardia. This is called an
'orthodromic reciprocating tachycardia' and it causes narrow QRS
complexes with P waves sometimes visible just after each QRS

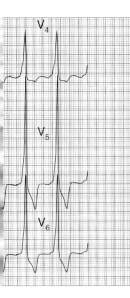

Fig. 1.42 Wolff–Parkinson–White syndrome

Note
- Sinus rhythm
- Short PR interval
- Wide QRS complex with initial delta wave
  (arrowed in inset)

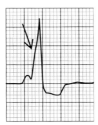

Delta wave in lead II

complex. Alternatively, depolarization can pass down the accessory pathway and retrogradely up the His bundle to cause an 'antidromic reciprocating tachycardia', in which the QRS complexes are broad and slurred, and P waves may or may not be seen.

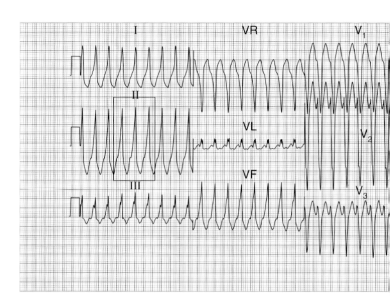

When a re-entry tachycardia occurs it may be difficult to decide whether it is supraventricular or ventricular in origin, unless an ECG is available that shows WPW conduction in sinus rhythm (Fig. 1.43).

The Lown–Ganong–Levine (LGL) syndrome is due to an AV node bypass that connects the atrium to the His bundle. When re-entry occurs the QRS complexes remain narrow, with appearances similar to those of a junctional tachycardia. The tachycardias due to the WPW and LGL syndromes are grouped together under the term 'atrioventricular re-entry (AVRE) tachycardias'. They are discussed further in Chapter 3.

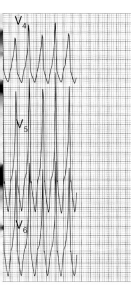

Fig. 1.43 Re-entry tachycardia

Note
- No P waves
- Broad complex tachycardia at 200/min
- Delta wave (arrowed in inset) suggests WPW syndrome

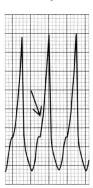

Delta wave in lead II

Atrial tachycardia and atrial flutter
Re-entry within the atrial muscle causes a tachycardia characterized by P waves with a shape different from that of those related to sinus rhythm. The PR interval is usually short (Fig. 1.44). Atrial tachycardia can also result from enhanced automaticity.

Atrial flutter is an organized atrial tachycardia, due to re-entry through a small circuit within the atrial muscle (Fig. 1.45).

Atrial fibrillation
In atrial fibrillation, 'flutter-like' waves sometimes appear intermittently and these depend on re-entry through circuits of varying lengths. 'Flutter fibrillation' behaves clinically like atrial fibrillation (Fig. 1.46).

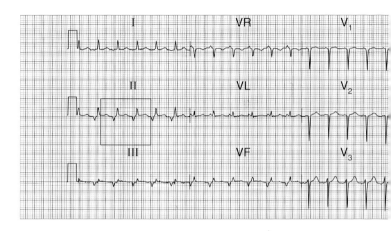

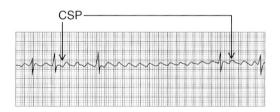

Fig. 1.45 Atrial flutter with carotid sinus pressure

Note
- Atrial flutter with 2:1 block
- Carotid sinus pressure (CSP) completely suppresses AV conduction, and there is no QRS complex for 3 seconds
- The 'flutter' waves become more obvious

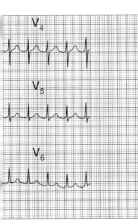

Fig. 1.44 Atrial tachycardia

Note
- P waves visible, but they are inverted in several leads
- Rate 140/min
- Normal QRS complexes

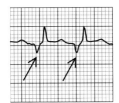

Inverted P waves in lead II

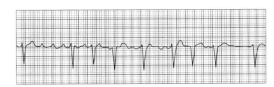

Fig. 1.46 Atrial fibrillation

Note
- Atrial fibrillation with a varying QRS complex rate but constant QRS configuration
- Initially, 'flutter' waves are present, but later these are replaced by the typical chaotic baseline of fibrillation
- This record is from lead V_1, which often shows atrial activity best in cases of atrial fibrillation and flutter

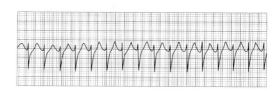

Fig. 1.47 AV nodal re-entry (junctional) tachycardia

Note
- No P waves can be seen
- QRS complexes are narrow and completely regular at 160/min

Junctional tachycardia

Junctional tachycardia occurs because of a congenital abnormality of the AV node, which allows re-entry to start and be sustained within the node itself. Atrial and ventricular activation are virtually simultaneous, so the P wave is hidden within the QRS complex (Fig. 1.47).

Junctional tachycardia is the most common form of paroxysmal tachycardia in young and middle-aged people, and it is often referred to as 'supraventricular tachycardia' or 'SVT'. In fact it is only one of the supraventricular tachycardias – properly speaking, sinus tachycardia, atrial tachycardia, atrial flutter and atrial fibrillation are all types of supraventricular tachycardia.

Because the AVRE tachycardias of the WPW and LGL syndromes involve the junctional region (i.e. the AV node and surrounding tissue), junctional tachycardias are most accurately called 'AV nodal re-entry' (AVNRE) tachycardias. However, the terms 'junctional tachycardia' and 'SVT' seem likely to persist in common usage.

Broad complex tachycardias

If a tachycardia shows a broad QRS complex, there are three possible causes:

- a supraventricular tachycardia with bundle branch block: here the mechanism of the tachycardia is that of the supraventricular rhythm, but conduction into the ventricles occurs through one bundle branch only

- re-entry tachycardia associated with the WPW syndrome
- ventricular tachycardia: here the arrhythmia may be due to re-entry through circuits within the Purkinje system, or may result from enhanced automaticity.

In ventricular tachycardia, the broad QRS complexes are of a constant configuration and are fairly regular if the re-entry pathway is constant (Fig. 1.48).

However, the re-entry pathway often varies slightly, causing variation in the shape of the QRS complexes and some irregularity in their timing. This is seen in its most extreme form in the torsade de pointes (TdP) variety of ventricular tachycardia (Fig. 1.49).

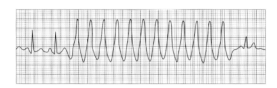

Fig. 1.48 Ventricular tachycardia

Note
- Two sinus beats are followed by ventricular tachycardia at 150/min
- The complexes are regular, with little variation in shape
- Sinus rhythm is then restored

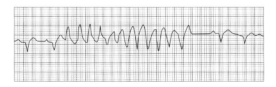

Fig. 1.49 Ventricular tachycardia (torsade de pointes)

Note
- Two sinus beats are followed by ventricular tachycardia
- The complexes initially point upwards, but then become inverted and the QRS complex rate is variable

Differentiation between re-entry and enhanced automaticity

Except in the case of the pre-excitation syndromes, there is no certain way of distinguishing from the surface ECG between a tachycardia due to enhanced automaticity and one due to re-entry. In general, however, tachycardias that follow or are terminated by extrasystoles, and those that can be initiated or inhibited by appropriately timed intracardiac pacing impulses, are likely to be due to re-entry (Figs 1.50 and 1.51).

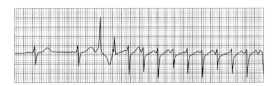

Fig. 1.50 Atrial tachycardia

Note
- After two sinus beats there is one ventricular extrasystole, and then a narrow complex that is probably supraventricular
- Atrial tachycardia is induced
- P waves are visible at the end of the T wave of the preceding beat

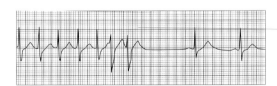

Fig. 1.51 Junctional tachycardia

Note
- Five beats of junctional tachycardia at 150/min are followed by two ventricular extrasystoles.
- These interrupt the tachycardia, and sinus rhythm is restored

The differentiation between tachycardias caused by enhanced automaticity and those caused by re-entry does not affect the choice of treatment.

THE QRS COMPLEX

Abnormalities of the QRS complex will be covered in later chapters, but since this is a 'revision' course it is worth remembering that there are three possible QRS abnormalities:

- The R waves may be too tall and the S waves too deep. This can be seen in normal people (see Ch. 2) or in ventricular hypertrophy (see Ch. 6).
- The QRS complex may be too wide, i.e. its duration may exceed the upper limit of 120 ms. This may result from bundle branch block (right or left) or a ventricular origin of depolarization.
- There may be Q waves. Small and narrow Q waves may result from septal depolarization that is initially from left to right (Fig. 1.52).

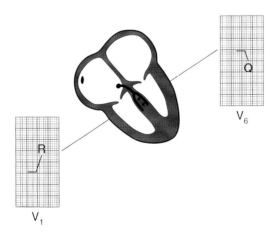

Fig. 1.52 Septal depolarization

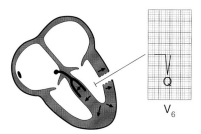

Fig. 1.53 Myocardial infarction

'Septal' Q waves are normal (see Ch. 2), but deeper or wider Q waves indicate a myocardial infarction. They occur because a lead over an electrical 'window' due to an infarction 'sees' depolarization moving away in all directions (Fig. 1.53). Infarction patterns are described in Chapter 4.

The ST segment and the T wave

The ST segment should be isoelectric, which means it should be at the same level as the ECG trace between beats (T wave to the next P wave). A raised ST segment can be a normal variant (see Ch. 2) or may indicate an acute myocardial infarction or pericarditis (see Ch. 4). A depressed ST segment may be due to ischaemia (see Ch. 4) or digoxin therapy (see Ch. 6).

The most important thing to remember about the T wave is in which leads it may be inverted in normal people:

- VR
- V_1 and sometimes V_2
- other chest leads in black people
- III, provided it is upright in VF.

These variations will be described in Chapter 2.

T wave inversion in other leads may be associated with:

- bundle branch block
- ventricular origin of depolarization
- ischaemia
- ventricular hypertrophy
- drugs.

A prolonged QT interval may be associated with:

- electrolyte disturbance
- drugs
- a congenital abnormality.

Peaked T waves are often normal, but can be due to hyperkalaemia.

2
The ECG in healthy people

THE RANGE OF NORMALITY IN THE ECG

For the purposes of this chapter, we shall assume that the subject from whom the ECG was recorded is asymptomatic, and that physical examination has revealed no abnormalities. We need to consider the range of normality of the ECG, but of course we cannot escape from the fact that not all disease causes symptoms or abnormal signs, and a subject who appears healthy may not be so and may therefore have an abnormal ECG. In particular, individuals who present for 'screening' may well have symptoms about which they have not consulted a doctor, so it cannot be assumed that an ECG obtained through a screening programme has come from a healthy subject.

The range of normality in the ECG is therefore debatable. We first have to consider the variations in the ECG that we can expect to find in completely healthy people, and then we can think about the significance of ECGs that are undoubtedly 'abnormal'.

ACCEPTABLE VARIATIONS IN THE NORMAL ECG

The normal cardiac rhythm

Sinus rhythm is the only normal sustained rhythm. In young people the R–R interval is reduced (that is, the heart rate is increased) during inspiration, and this is called sinus arrhythmia (Fig. 2.1). When sinus arrhythmia is marked, it may mimic an atrial arrhythmia. However, in sinus arrhythmia each P–QRS–T complex is normal, and it is only the interval between them that changes.

Sinus arrhythmia becomes less marked with increasing age of the subject, and is lost in conditions such as diabetic autonomic neuropathy. This is because vagus nerve function is impaired.

The heart rate

There is no such thing as a normal heart, and the terms 'tachycardia' and 'bradycardia' should be used with care. There is no point at which a high heart rate in sinus rhythm has to be called 'sinus tachycardia' and there is no upper limit for 'sinus bradycardia'. Nevertheless, unexpectedly fast or slow rates do need an explanation.

Sinus tachycardia
The ECG in Figure 2.2 was recorded from a young woman who complained of a fast heart rate. She had no other symptoms but was anxious. There were no other abnormalities on examination, and her blood count and thyroid function tests were normal.

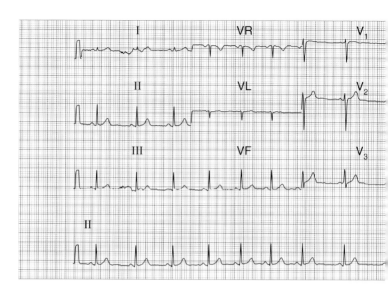

Fig. 2.2 Sinus tachycardia

Note
- Normal P–QRS–T waves
- R–R interval 600 ms
- Heart rate 120/min

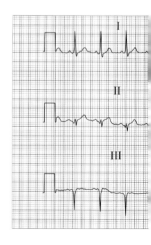

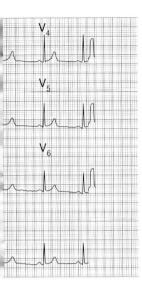

Fig. 2.1 Sinus arrhythmia

Note
- Marked variation in R–R interval
- Constant PR interval
- Constant shape of P wave and QRS complex

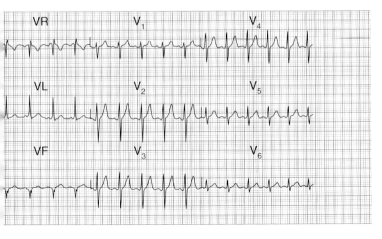

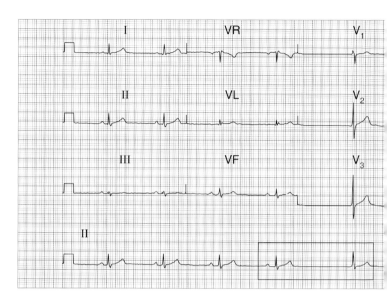

The possible causes of sinus rhythm with a fast heart rate are:

- pain, fright, exercise
- hypovolaemia
- myocardial infarction
- heart failure
- pulmonary embolism
- obesity
- lack of physical fitness
- pregnancy
- thyrotoxicosis
- anaemia
- beri-beri
- CO_2 retention
- autonomic neuropathy
- drugs:
  - sympathomimetics
  - salbutamol (including by inhalation)
  - caffeine
  - atropine.

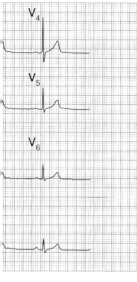

Fig. 2.3 Sinus bradycardia

Note
- Sinus rhythm
- Rate 44/min
- One junctional escape beat

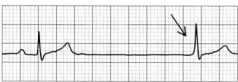

Junctional escape beat

Sinus bradycardia

The ECG in Figure 2.3 was recorded from a young professional footballer. His heart rate was 44/min, and at one point the sinus rate became so slow that a junctional escape beat appeared.

The possible causes of sinus rhythm with a slow heart rate are:

- physical fitness
- vasovagal attacks
- sick sinus syndrome
- acute myocardial infarction, especially inferior
- hypothyroidism
- hypothermia

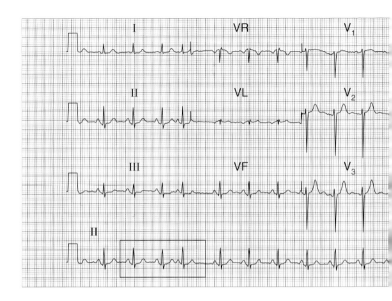

- obstructive jaundice
- raised intracranial pressure
- drugs:
  - beta-blockers (including eye drops for glaucoma)
  - verapamil
  - digoxin.

Extrasystoles

Supraventricular extrasystoles, either atrial or junctional (AV nodal), occur commonly in normal people and are of no significance (Fig. 2.4). Atrial extrasystoles have an abnormal P wave; in junctional extrasystoles, either there is no P wave or the P wave may follow the QRS complex.

Ventricular extrasystoles are also commonly seen in normal ECGs (Fig. 2.5).

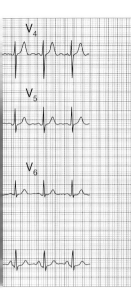

Fig. 2.4 Supraventricular extrasystole

Note
- In supraventricular extrasystoles the QRS complex and the T wave are the same as in the sinus beat
- The fourth beat has an abnormal P wave and therefore an atrial origin

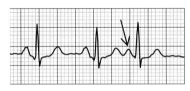

Early abnormal P wave

The P wave

In sinus rhythm, the P wave is normally upright in all leads except VR. When the QRS complex is predominantly downward in lead VL, the P wave may also be inverted (Fig. 2.6).

In patients with dextrocardia (Fig. 2.7) the P wave is inverted in lead I. In practice this is more often seen if the limb leads have been wrongly attached, but dextrocardia can be recognized if leads V_5 and V_6, which normally 'look at' the left ventricle, show a predominantly downward QRS complex.

If the ECG of a patient with dextrocardia is repeated with the limb leads reversed, and the chest leads are placed on the right side of the chest in a position corresponding to those normally used on the left side, the ECG becomes like that of a normal patient (Fig. 2.8).

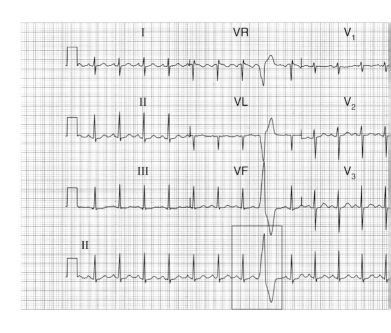

Fig. 2.6 Normal ECG

Note
- In both VR and VL the P wave is inverted, and the QRS complex is predominantly downward

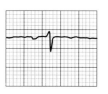

Inverted P wave
in lead VL

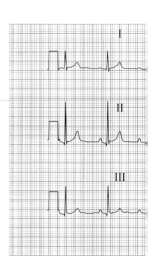

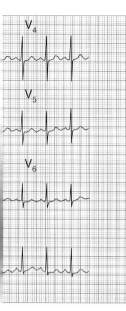

Fig. 2.5 Ventricular extrasystole

Note
- Sinus rhythm, with one ventricular extrasystole
- Extrasystole has a wide and abnormal QRS complex and an abnormal T wave

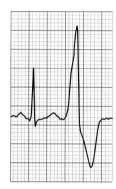

Ventricular extrasystole

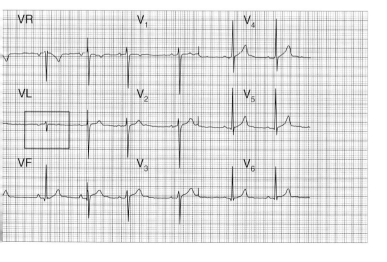

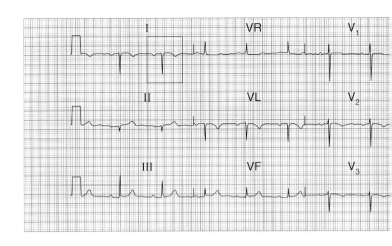

Fig. 2.8 Dextrocardia, leads reversed

Note
- P wave in lead I upright
- QRS complex upright in lead I
- Typical left ventricular complex in lead V_6

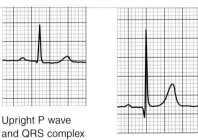

Upright P wave
and QRS complex
in lead I

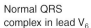

Normal QRS
complex in lead V_6

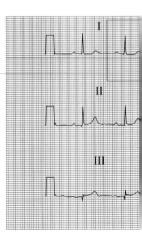

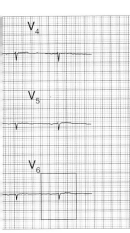

Fig. 2.7 Dextrocardia

Note
- Inverted P wave in lead I
- No left ventricular complexes seen in leads V_5, V_6

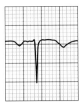

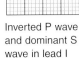

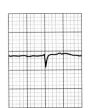

Inverted P wave and dominant S wave in lead I

Persistent S wave in lead V_6

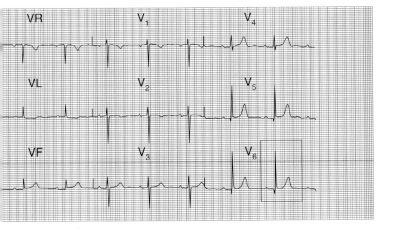

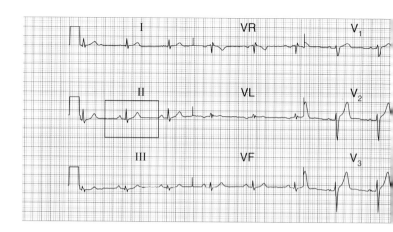

The PR interval

In sinus rhythm, the PR interval is constant and the normal range is 120–220 ms (3–5 small squares of ECG paper) (Fig. 2.9).

A PR interval of less than 120 ms suggests pre-excitation, and a PR interval of longer than 220 ms is due to first degree block. Both of these 'abnormalities' are seen in normal people, and will be discussed further in Chapter 3.

The QRS complex

The cardiac axis

There is a fairly wide range of normality in the direction of the cardiac axis. In most people the QRS complex is tallest in lead II, but in leads I and III the QRS complex is also predominantly upright (i.e. the R wave is greater than the S wave) (Fig. 2.10).

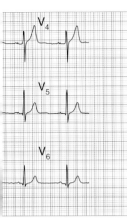

Fig. 2.9 Normal ECG

Note
- PR interval 170 ms
- PR interval constant in all leads
- Notched P wave in lead V_5 is often normal

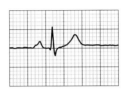

PR interval
170 ms in lead II

The cardiac axis is still perfectly normal when the R wave and S wave are equal in lead I: this is common in tall people (Fig. 2.11).

When the S wave is greater than the R wave in lead I, right axis deviation is present. However, this is very common in perfectly normal people. The ECG in Figure 2.12 is from a professional footballer.

It is common for the S wave to be greater than the R wave in lead III, and the cardiac axis can still be considered normal when the S wave equals the R wave in lead II. These patterns are common in fat people and during pregnancy (Fig. 2.13).

When the depth of the S wave exceeds the height of the R wave in lead II, left axis deviation is present (see Fig 3.21).

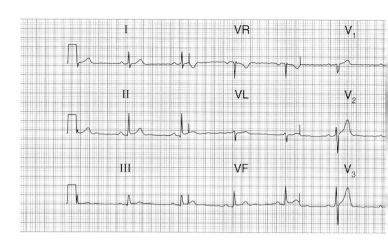

Fig. 2.11 Normal ECG

Note
- This record shows the 'rightward' limit of normality of the cardiac axis
- R and S waves equal in lead I

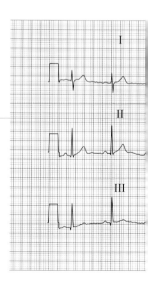

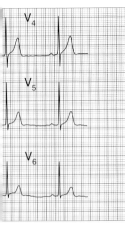

Fig. 2.10 Normal ECG

Note
- QRS complex upright in leads I, II, III
- R wave tallest in lead II

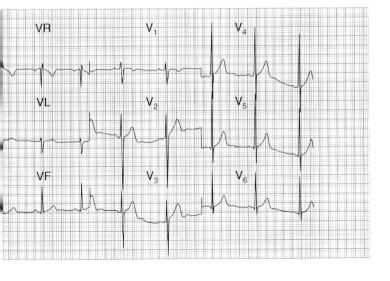

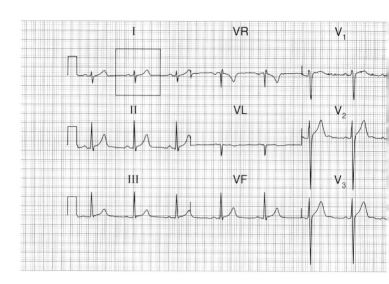

Fig. 2.13 Normal ECG

Note
- This shows the 'leftward' limit of normality of the cardiac axis
- S wave equals R wave in lead II
- S wave greater than R wave in lead III

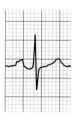

S wave = R wave in lead II

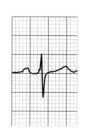

S wave > R wave in lead III

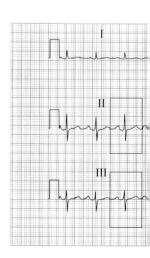

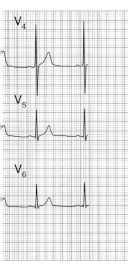

Fig. 2.12 ?Normal ECG

Note
- Right axis deviation: S wave greater than R wave in lead I
- Upright QRS complexes in leads II, III

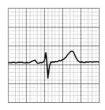

Dominant S wave in lead I

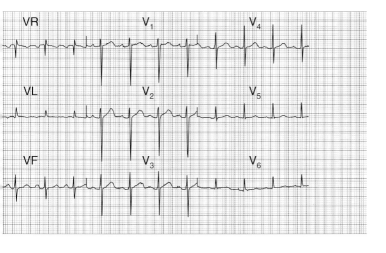

The size of R and S waves in the chest leads
In lead V_1 there should be a small R wave and a deep S wave, and the balance between the two should change progressively from V_1–V_6. In lead V_6 there should be a tall R wave and no S wave (Fig. 2.14).

Typically the 'transition point', when the R and S waves are equal, is seen in lead III or V_4 but there is quite a lot of variation. Figure 2.15 shows an ECG in which the transition point is somewhere between leads V_3 and V_4.

Figure 2.16 shows an ECG with a transition point between leads V_4 and V_5.

Figure 2.17 shows an ECG with a transition point between leads V_2 and V_3.

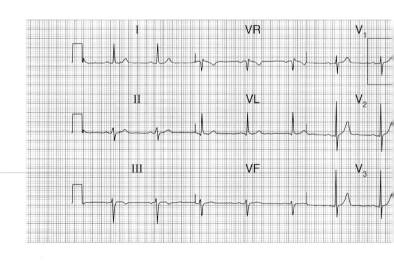

The 'transition' is typically seen in lead V_5 or even V_6 in patients with chronic lung disease (see Ch. 5), and this is called 'clockwise rotation'. A similar ECG pattern may be seen in patients with an abnormal chest shape, particularly when depression of the sternum shifts the mediastinum to the left although in this case the term 'clockwise rotation' is not used. The patient from whom the ECG in Figure 2.18 was recorded had mediastinal shift.

Occasionally the ECG of a totally normal subject will show a 'dominant' R wave (i.e. the height of the R wave exceeds the depth of the S wave) in lead V_1. There will thus, effectively, be no transition point. The ECG in Figure 2.19 was recorded from a healthy footballer with a normal heart. However, a dominant R wave in lead V_1 is usually due to either right ventricular hypertrophy (see Ch. 4) or a true posterior infarction (see Ch. 3).

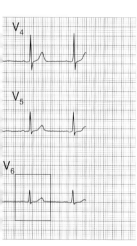

Fig. 2.14 Normal ECG

Note

- Lead V_1 shows a predominantly downward complex, with the S wave greater than the R wave
- Lead V_6 shows an upright complex, with a dominant R wave and a tiny S wave

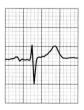
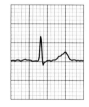

S wave > R wave
in lead V_1

Dominant R wave
in lead V_6

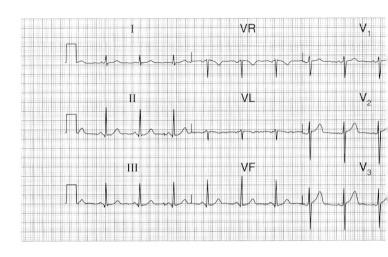

Fig. 2.16 Normal ECG

Note
- Dominant S wave in lead V_4
- R wave just bigger than S wave in lead V_5

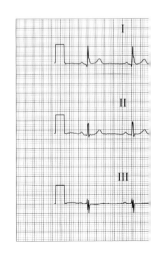

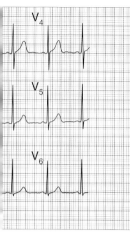

Fig. 2.15 Normal ECG

Note
- In lead V_3 there is a dominant S wave
- In lead V_4 there is a dominant R wave
- The transition point is between leads V_3 and V_4

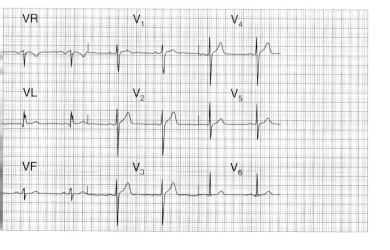

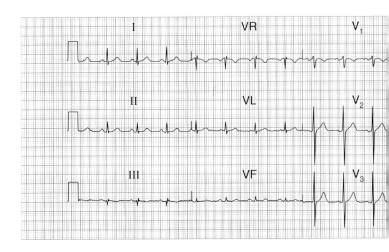

Fig. 2.18
Mediastinal shift

Note
- 'Abnormal' ECG, but a normal heart
- Shift of the mediastinum means the transition point is under lead V_6
- Ventricular complexes are shown in leads round the left side of the chest, in positions V_7–V_9

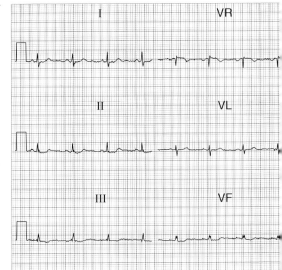

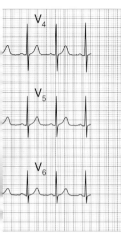

Fig. 2.17 Normal ECG

Note
- Dominant S wave in lead V_2
- Dominant R wave in lead V_3
- The transition point is between leads V_2 and V_3

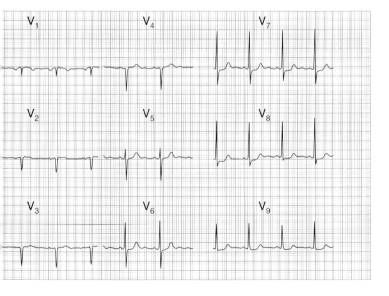

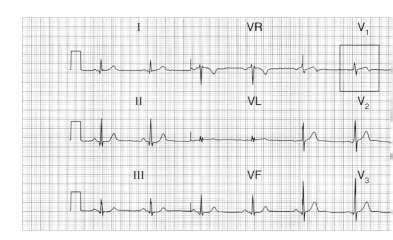

   Although the balance between the height of the R wave and
the depth of the S wave is significant for identifying a degree
of cardiac axis deviation, and for the identification of right
ventricular hypertrophy, the absolute height of the R wave
provides little useful information. Provided that the ECG is
properly calibrated (1 mV causes 1 centimetre of vertical deflection
on the ECG), the limits for the sizes of the R and S waves in
normal subjects are usually said to be:

- 25 mm for the R wave in lead V_5 or V_6
- 25 mm for the S wave in lead V_1 or V_2
- Sum of R wave in lead V_5 or V_6 plus S wave in lead V_1 or V_2
  should be less than 35 mm.

However, R waves taller than 25 mm are commonly seen in leads
V_5–V_6 in fit and thin young people, and are perfectly normal.
These 'limits' are not helpful. The ECGs in Figures 2.20 and 2.21
were both recorded from fit young men with normal hearts.

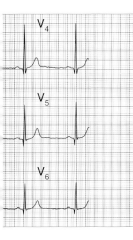

Fig. 2.19 Normal ECG

Note
- Dominant R waves in lead V_1

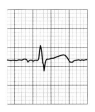

Dominant R wave in lead V_1

The width of the QRS complex

The QRS complex should be less than 120 ms in duration (i.e. less than 3 small squares) in all leads. If it is longer than this, then either the ventricles have been depolarized from a ventricular rather than a supraventricular focus (i.e. a ventricular rhythm is present), or there is an abnormality of conduction within the ventricle. The latter is most commonly due to bundle branch block. An RSR^1 pattern, resembling that of right bundle branch block (RBBB) but with a narrow QRS complex, is sometimes called 'partial right bundle branch block' and is a normal variant (Figs 2.22 and 2.23).

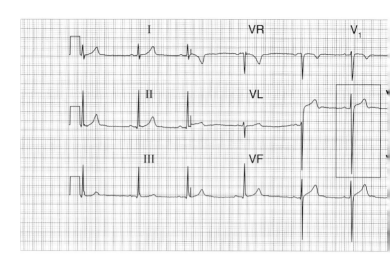

Fig. 2.21 Normal ECG

Note
• R wave in lead V_5 is 42 mm

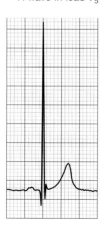

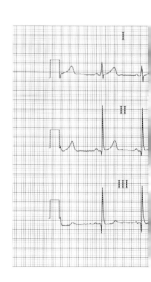

R wave > 25 mm
in lead V_5

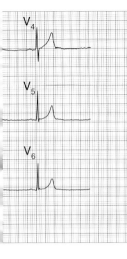

Fig. 2.20 Normal ECG

Note
- S wave in lead V_2 is 36 mm

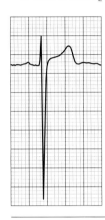

S wave > 25 mm in lead V_2

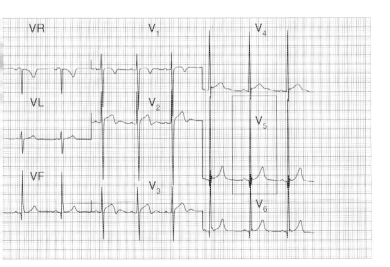

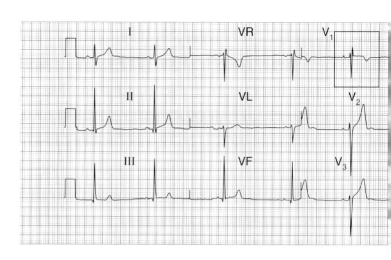

Fig. 2.23 Normal ECG

Note
- RSR¹ pattern in lead V₁
- Notched S wave in lead V₂
- QRS complex duration 100 ms
- Partial RBBB pattern

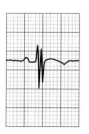

RSR¹ pattern in
lead V₁

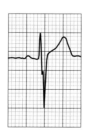

Notched S wave
in lead V₂

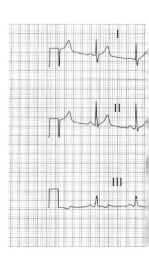

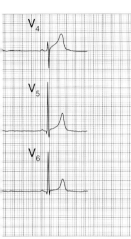

Fig. 2.22 Normal ECG

Note
- RSR^1 pattern in lead V$_2$
- QRS complex duration 100 ms
- Partial RBBB pattern

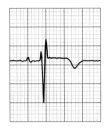

RSR^1 pattern and
QRS complex 100 ms
in lead V$_1$

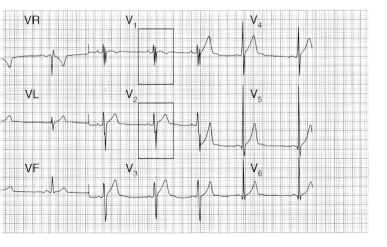

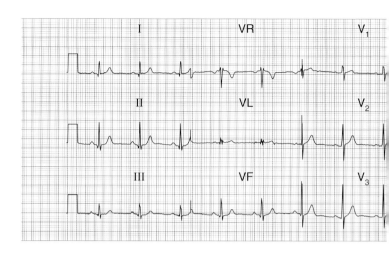

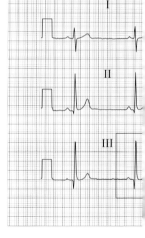

Fig. 2.25 Normal ECG

Note
- Narrow but quite deep Q wave in lead III
- Smaller Q wave in lead VF

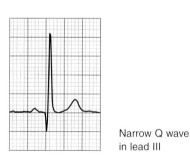

Narrow Q wave
in lead III

Q waves

The normal depolarization of the interventricular septum from left to right (see Fig. 1.52) causes a small 'septal' Q wave in any of leads II, VL, or V_5–V_6. Septal Q waves are usually less than 3 mm deep and less than 1 mm across (Fig. 2.24).

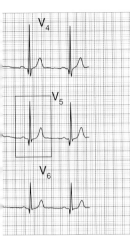

Fig. 2.24 Normal ECG

Note
- 'Septal' Q waves in leads I, II, V_4–V_6

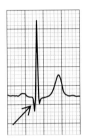

Septal Q wave in lead V_5

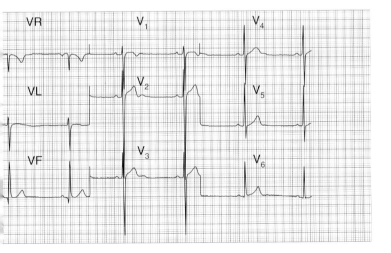

A small Q wave is also common in lead III in normal people: it is then always narrow but can be more than 3 mm deep. Occasionally there will be a similar Q wave in lead VF (Fig. 2.25). These 'normal' Q waves become much less deep, and may disappear altogether, on deep inspiration.

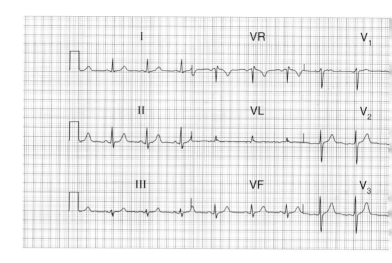

The ST segment

The ST segment (the part of the ECG between the S wave and the T wave) should be horizontal and 'isoelectric', which means that it should be at the same level as the baseline of the record between the end of the T wave and the next P wave. However, in the chest leads the ST segment often slopes upwards and is not easy to define (Fig. 2.26).

An elevation of the ST segment is the hallmark of an acute myocardial infarction (see Ch. 4), and depression of the ST segment can indicate ischaemia or the effect of digoxin. However, it is perfectly normal for the ST segment to be elevated following an S wave in leads V_2–V_5. This is sometimes called a 'high take-off ST segment'. The ECGs in Figures 2.27 and 2.28 were recorded from perfectly healthy young men.

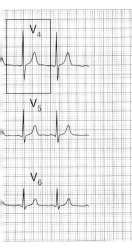

Fig. 2.26 Normal ECG

Note
- ST segment is isoelectric but slopes upwards in leads V_2–V_5

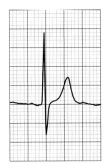

Upward-sloping ST segment in lead V_4

Depression of the ST segment is not uncommon in normal people, and is then called 'nonspecific'. ST segment depression in lead III but not VF is likely to be nonspecific (Fig. 2.29). Nonspecific ST segment depression should not be more than 2 mm (Fig. 2.30), and the segment often slopes upward. Horizontal ST segment depression of more than 2 mm indicates ischaemia (see Ch. 4).

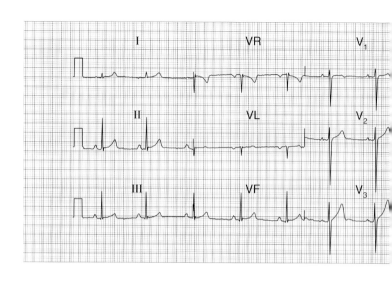

Fig. 2.28 Normal ECG

Note
- Marked ST segment elevation in lead V_3 follows an S wave

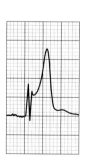

High take-off ST segment in lead V_3

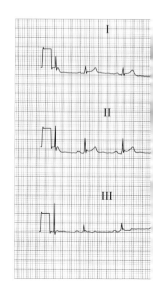

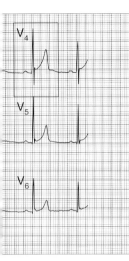

Fig. 2.27 Normal ECG

Note

- In lead V_4 there is an S wave followed by a raised ST segment. This is a 'high take-off' ST segment

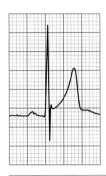

High take-off ST segment in lead V_4

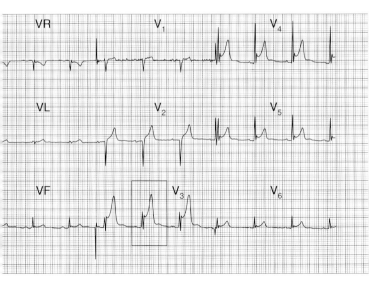

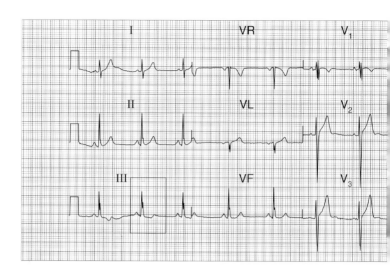

Fig. 2.30 Possibly normal ECG

Note

- ST segment depression of 1 mm in leads V₃–V₆
- In a patient with chest pain this would be suspicious of ischaemia but, particularly in women, such changes can be 'nonspecific'

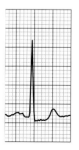

Nonspecific ST segment depression in lead V₅

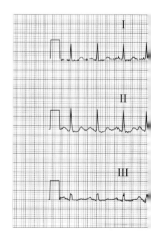

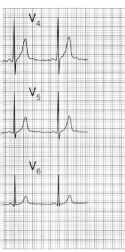

Fig. 2.29 Normal ECG

Note
- ST segment depression in lead III but not VF
- Biphasic T wave (i.e. initially inverted but then upright) in lead III but not VF
- Partial RBBB pattern

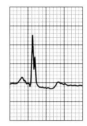

ST segment depression and biphasic T wave in lead III

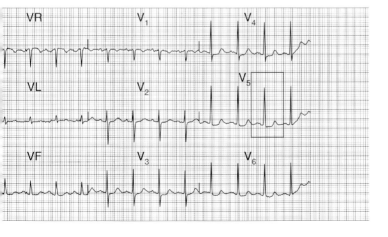

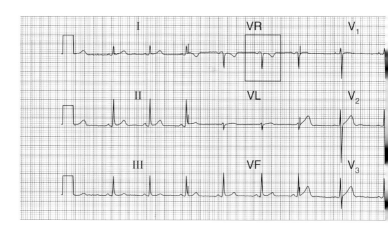

Fig. 2.32 Normal ECG

Note

- Small Q wave in lead III but not VF
- Inverted T wave in lead III but upright T wave in VF
- Inverted T wave in lead V₁

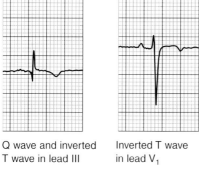

Q wave and inverted
T wave in lead III

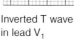

Inverted T wave
in lead V₁

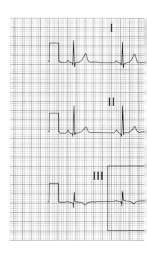

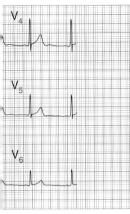

Fig. 2.31 Normal ECG

Note
- T wave is inverted in VR but is upright in all other leads

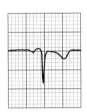

Inverted T wave in lead VR

The T wave

In a normal ECG the T wave is always inverted in lead VR but is usually upright in all the other leads (Fig. 2.31).

The T wave is often inverted in lead III but not VF. However, its inversion in lead III is reversed on deep inspiration (Figs 2.32 and 2.33). T wave inversion is also common in lead V₁.

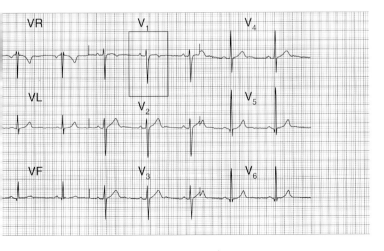

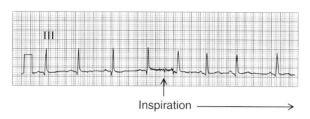

Inspiration ⟶

Fig. 2.33 Normal ECG during inspiration

Note
- ECG recorded from same patient as in Figure 2.32, but during deep inspiration
- Q wave in lead III disappears
- T wave becomes upright

T wave inversion in lead VL as well as in VR can be normal, particularly if the P wave in lead VL is inverted. The ECG in Figure 2.34 was recorded from a completely healthy young woman.

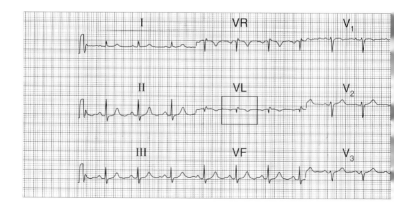

T wave inversion in leads V_2–V_3 as well as in V_1 occurs in pulmonary embolism and in right ventricular hypertrophy (see Chs 4 and 5) but it can be a normal variant. This is particularly true in black people. The ECG in Figure 2.35 was recorded from a healthy young white man, and that shown in Figure 2.36 from a young black professional footballer. The ECG in Figure 2.37 was recorded from a middle-aged black woman with rather nonspecific chest pain, whose coronary arteries and left ventricle were shown to be entirely normal on catheterization.

Generalized flattening of the T waves with a normal QT interval is best described as 'nonspecific'. In a patient without symptoms and whose heart is clinically normal, the finding has little prognostic significance. This was the case in the patient whose ECG is shown in Figure 2.38. In patients with symptoms suggestive of cardiovascular disease, however, such an ECG would require further investigation.

Peaked T waves are one of the features of hyperkalaemia, but they can also be very prominent in healthy people (Fig. 2.39).

The T wave is the most variable part of the ECG. It may become inverted in some leads simply by hyperventilation associated with anxiety.

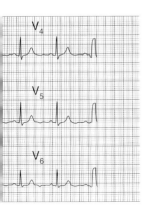

Fig. 2.34 Normal ECG

Note
- Inverted T waves in leads VR, VL
- Inverted P waves in leads VR, VL

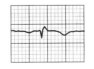

Inverted P and T waves
in lead VL

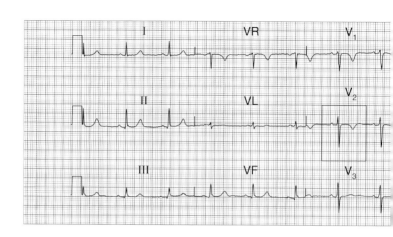

Fig. 2.36 Normal ECG, from a black man

Note
• T wave inversion in leads VR, V$_1$, V$_2$, V$_3$

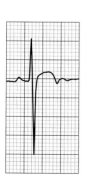

Inverted T wave in
lead V$_3$

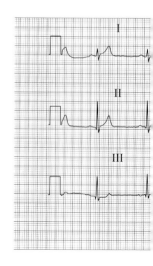

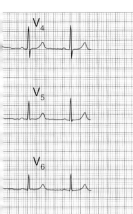

Fig. 2.35 Normal ECG

Note
- T wave inversion in leads VR, V_1, V_2
- Biphasic T wave in lead V_3

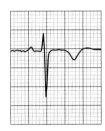

Inverted T wave in lead V_2

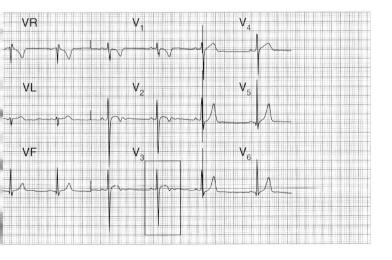

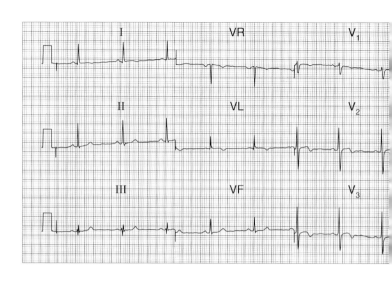

Fig. 2.38 Possibly normal ECG

Note
- Sinus rhythm
- Normal axis
- Normal QRS complexes
- T wave flattening in all chest leads
- T wave inversion in leads III, VF
- In an asymptomatic patient, these changes are not necessarily significant

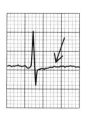

Flattened T wave in lead V₃

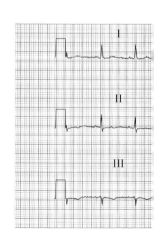

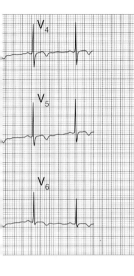

Fig. 2.37 Normal ECG, from a black woman

Note
- Sinus rhythm
- T wave inversion in lead VL and all chest leads
- Presumably a normal variant: coronary angiography and echocardiography were normal

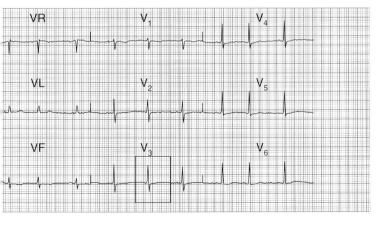

95

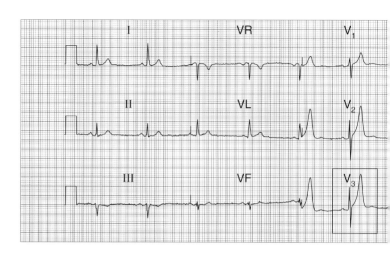

Fig. 2.40 Normal ECG

Note
- Prominent U waves following normal T waves in leads V_2–V_4

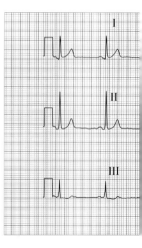

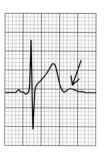

U wave in lead V_3

An extra hump on the end of the T wave, a 'U' wave, is characteristic of hypokalaemia. However, U waves are commonly seen in the anterior chest leads of normal ECGs (Fig. 2.40). It is thought that they represent repolarization of the papillary muscles. A U wave is probably only important if it follows a flat T wave.

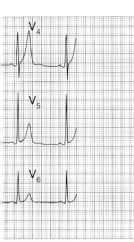

Fig. 2.39 Normal ECG

Note
- Sinus rhythm
- Normal axis
- Normal QRS complexes
- Very tall and peaked T waves

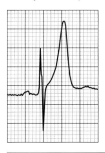

Tall peaked T wave in lead V$_3$

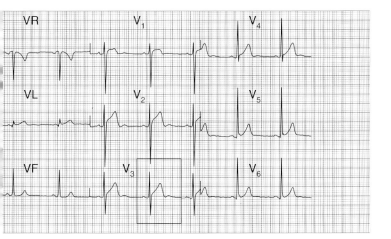

The QT interval

The QT interval (from the Q wave to the end of the T wave) varies with the heart rate, gender and time of day. There are several different ways of correcting for heart rate, but the simplest is Bazett's formula. In this, the corrected QT interval, QT$_c$, is calculated by:

97

$$QT_c = \frac{QT}{\sqrt{(R-R\ interval)}}$$

It is, however, uncertain whether QT_c has any greater clinical significance than the uncorrected QT interval. The normal QT interval is 340–430 ms, and whatever the rate, a QT interval > 450 ms is probably pathological.

THE ECG IN ATHLETES

Most of the normal variations discussed above are common in athletes. Below are listed some of the ECG features that might be considered abnormal in non-athletic subjects, but normal in athletes.

Variations in rhythm:

- Sinus bradycardia
- Marked sinus arrhythmia
- Junctional rhythm

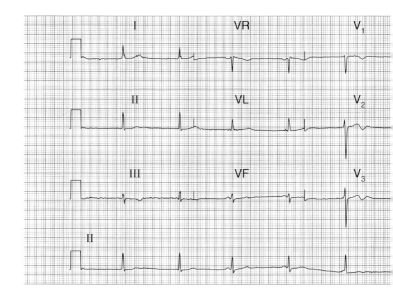

- 'Wandering' atrial pacemaker
- First degree block
- Wenckebach phenomenon
- Second degree block.

Variations in ECG pattern:

- Tall P waves
- Tall R waves and deep S waves
- Prominent septal Q waves
- Counterclockwise rotation
- Slight ST segment elevation
- Tall symmetrical T waves
- T wave inversion, especially in lateral leads
- Biphasic T waves
- Prominent U waves.

The ECGs in Figures 2.41, 2.42 and 2.43 were all recorded during the screening examinations of healthy young footballers.

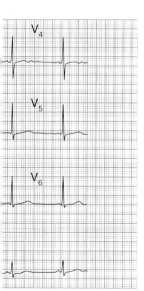

Fig. 2.41 Normal ECG

Note
- Heart rate 49/min
- Accelerated idionodal rhythm ('wandering pacemaker')
- Biphasic T wave in lead V_3
- Prominent U waves

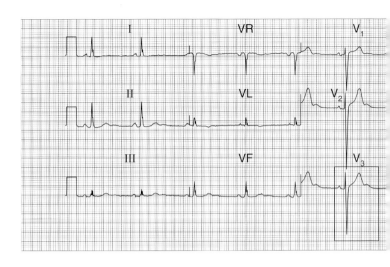

Fig. 2.43 Normal ECG

Note

- Sinus rhythm
- Left axis deviation
- Septal Q waves in leads V_5, V_6

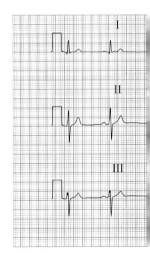

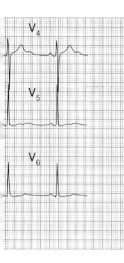

Fig. 2.42 Normal ECG

Note
- Heart rate 53/min
- Sinus rhythm
- Prominent U waves in leads V_2–V_5
- Inverted T waves in lead VL

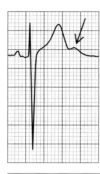

U wave in lead V_3

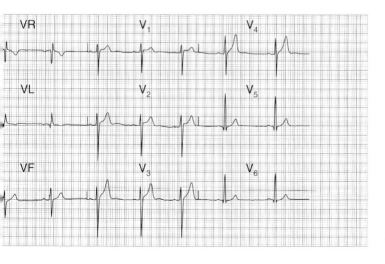

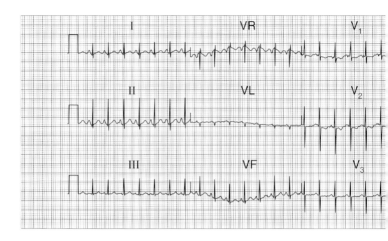

THE ECG IN CHILDREN

The normal heart rate in the first year of life is 140–160/min, falling slowly to about 80/min by puberty. Sinus arrhythmia is usually quite marked in children.

At birth, the muscle of the right ventricle is as thick as that of the left ventricle. The ECG of a normal child in the first year of life has a pattern that would indicate right ventricular hypertrophy in an adult. The ECG in Figure 2.44 was recorded from a normal child aged 1 month.

The changes suggestive of right ventricular hypertrophy disappear during the first few years of life. All the features other than the inverted T waves in leads V_1 and V_2 should have disappeared by the age of 2 years, and the adult pattern of the ECG should have developed by the age of 10 years. In general, if the infant ECG pattern persists beyond the age of 2 years, then right ventricular hypertrophy is indeed present. If the normal adult pattern is present in the first year of life, then left ventricular hypertrophy is present.

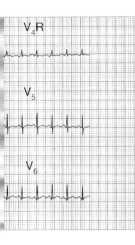

Fig. 2.44 Normal ECG, from a child 1 month old

Note
- Heart rate 170/min
- Sinus rhythm
- Normal axis
- Dominant R waves in lead V_1
- Inverted T waves in leads V_1, V_2
- Biphasic T waves in lead V_3
- Lead V_4R (a position on the chest equivalent to V_4, but on the right side) has been recorded instead of V_4

SPECIFIC ECG ABNORMALITIES IN HEALTHY PEOPLE

The ECG findings we have discussed so far can all be considered to be within the normal range. Certain findings are undoubtedly abnormal as far as the ECG is concerned, yet do occur in apparently healthy people.

The frequency with which abnormalities are detected depends on the population studied: most abnormalities are found least often in healthy young people recruited to the armed services, and become progressively more common in populations of increasing age. An exception to this rule is that frequent ventricular extrasystoles are very common in pregnancy. The frequency of right and left bundle branch block (RBBB and LBBB) has been found to be 0.3% and 0.1% respectively in populations of young service recruits, but in older working populations these abnormalities have been detected in 2% and 0.7% respectively of apparently healthy people.

Table 2.1 Prevalence of the more common ECG abnormalities in 18 000 civil servants (after Rose et al 1978 British Heart Journal 40: 636–643)

ECG abnormality	Rate of abnormality per 1000 individuals in age range		
	40–49 years	50–59 years	60–64 years
Frequent ventricular extrasystoles	8	14	26
Atrial fibrillation	2	4	11
Left axis deviation	23	32	49
First degree block	18	26	33
Left bundle branch block	9	16	31
Abnormal T wave inversion	9	54	76
WPW syndrome	0.3	0.2	0

Table 2.1 shows the frequency with which the more common ECG abnormalities were encountered in a large survey of civil servants. All the abnormalities, except the Wolff–Parkinson–White (WPW) syndrome, which is congenital (see Ch.1), were found more frequently with increasing age. The survey was of a working population, but some individuals had symptoms of heart disease and of course these were more common in the older age group. This suggests that the various abnormalities are all indicators of heart disease. This sort of survey shows how difficult it is to define the precise range of 'normality' in the ECG.

WHAT TO DO

When an apparently healthy subject has an ECG record that appears abnormal, the most important thing is not to cause unnecessary alarm. There are four questions to ask:

1. Does the ECG really come from that individual? If so, is he or she really asymptomatic and are the findings of the physical examination really normal?
2. Is the ECG really abnormal or is it within the normal range?

3. If the ECG is indeed abnormal, what are the implications for the patient?
4. What further investigations are needed?

The range of normality

Normal variations in the P waves, QRS complexes and T waves have been described in detail. T wave changes usually give the most trouble in terms of ECG interpretation, because changes in repolarization occur in many different circumstances, and in any individual variations in T wave morphology can occur from day to day. Below are listed some of the ECG patterns that can be accepted as normal in healthy patients, and some that must be regarded with suspicion.

Always normal:

- Sinus arrhythmia
- Supraventricular extrasystoles
- Incomplete RBBB
- 'High take-off' ST segment
- T wave inversion in lead III but not VF
- T wave inversion in leads VR and V_1.

Not necessarily indicative of heart disease:

- Ventricular extrasystoles
- Left or right axis deviation
- RBBB
- T wave inversion in leads other than III, VR and V_1
- Nonspecific ST segment changes.

The prognosis of patients with an abnormal ECG

In general, the prognosis is related to the patient's clinical history and to the findings on physical examination, rather than to the ECG. An abnormal ECG is much more significant in a patient with symptoms and signs of heart disease than it is in a truly healthy subject. In the absence of any other evidence of heart disease, the prognosis of an individual with one of the more common ECG abnormalities is as follows.

Conduction defects
First degree block (especially when the PR interval is only slightly prolonged) has little effect on prognosis. Second and third degree block indicate heart disease and the prognosis is worse, though the congenital form of complete block is less serious than the acquired form in adults.

Left anterior hemiblock has a good prognosis, as does RBBB. The presence of LBBB in the absence of other manifestations of cardiac disease is associated with about a 30% increase in the risk of death compared with that of individuals with a normal ECG. The risk of death doubles if a subject known to have a normal ECG suddenly develops LBBB, even if there are no symptoms. Bifascicular block seldom progresses to complete block, but is always an indication of underlying heart disease and the prognosis is therefore relatively poor.

Arrhythmias
Supraventricular extrasystoles are of no importance whatsoever. Ventricular extrasystoles are almost universal, but when frequent or multiform they indicate populations with an increased risk of death, presumably because in a proportion of people they indicate subclinical heart disease. The increased risk to an individual is, however, minimal and there is no evidence that treating ventricular extrasystoles prolongs survival.

Atrial fibrillation is frequently the result of rheumatic or ischaemic heart disease or cardiomyopathy, and the prognosis is then relatively poor. In about one third of individuals with atrial fibrillation no cardiac disease can be demonstrated, but in such people the risk of death is increased by three or four times, and the risk of stroke is increased perhaps tenfold, compared with people of the same age whose hearts are in sinus rhythm.

Further investigations
Complex and expensive investigations are seldom justified in asymptomatic patients whose hearts are clinically normal but who have been found to have an abnormal ECG.

A chest X-ray should probably be taken in patients with bundle branch block or atrial fibrillation, to provide an accurate estimate of heart size. Since LBBB may indicate a dilated cardiomyopathy, an echocardiogram can be recorded to assess left ventricular function. Echocardiography may be diagnostically useful but therapeutically unhelpful if anterior T wave inversion raises the possibility of hypertrophic cardiomyopathy.

Patients with frequent ventricular extrasystoles may merit a chest X-ray and the measurement of their haemoglobin level, but nothing else.

In patients with atrial fibrillation, an echocardiogram is useful for defining or excluding structural abnormalities, and for studying left ventricular function. An echocardiogram is indicated if there is anything that might suggest rheumatic heart disease. Since atrial fibrillation can be the only manifestation of thyrotoxicosis, thyroid function must be checked. Atrial fibrillation may also be the result of alcoholism and this may be denied by the patient, so it may be fair to check liver function.

Table 2.2, overleaf, shows investigations that should be considered for various cardiac rhythms and indicates which underlying diseases may be present.

Treatment of asymptomatic ECG abnormalities

It is always the patient who should be treated, not the ECG. The prognosis of patients with complete heart block is improved by permanent pacing, but that of patients with other degrees of block is not. Ventricular extrasystoles should not be treated because of the risk of the pro-arrhythmic effects of antiarrhythmic drugs. Atrial fibrillation need not be treated if the ventricular rate is reasonable, but anticoagulation must be considered in all cases. In the case of patients with valve disease and atrial fibrillation, however, anticoagulant treatment is essential.

Table 2.2 Investigations in apparently healthy people with an abnormal ECG

ECG appearance	Investigation	Diagnosis to be excluded
Sinus tachycardia	Thyroid function	Thyrotoxicosis
	Haemoglobin	Anaemia
	Chest X-ray	Changes in heart size
		Heart failure
	Echocardiogram	Systolic dysfunction
Sinus bradycardia	Thyroid function	Myxoedema
Right bundle branch block	Chest X-ray	Heart size
	Echocardiogram	Lung disease
		Atrial septal defect
Left bundle branch block	Chest X-ray	Heart size
	Echocardiogram	Aortic stenosis
		Cardiomyopathy
		Ischaemia
T wave abnormalities	Electrolytes	High or low potassium or calcium
	Echocardiogram	Ventricular systolic dysfunction
		Hypertrophic cardiomyopathy
	Exercise test	Ischaemia
Atrial fibrillation	Thyroid function	Thyrotoxicosis
	Liver function	Alcoholism
	Chest X-ray	Valve disease,
	Echocardiogram	ventricular and left atrial dimensions
		Myxoma

3

The ECG in patients with palpitations and syncope

INTRODUCTION

The ECG is of paramount importance for the diagnosis of arrhythmias. Many arrhythmias are not noticed by the patient, but sometimes they cause symptoms. These symptoms are often transient, and the patient may be completely well at the time he or she consults a doctor. Obtaining an ECG during a symptomatic episode is then the only certain way of making a diagnosis, but as always the history and physical examination are also extremely important. The main purpose of the history and examination is to

109

help decide whether a patient's symptoms could be the result of an arrhythmia, and whether the patient has a cardiac or other disease that may cause an arrhythmia.

THE CLINICAL HISTORY

Palpitations

'Palpitations' mean different things to different patients, but a general definition would be 'an awareness of the heartbeat'. Arrhythmias, fast or slow, can cause poor organ perfusion and so lead to syncope (a word used to describe all sorts of collapse), breathlessness and angina. Some rhythms can be recognized from a patient's description, such as:

- A patient recognizes sinus tachycardia because it feels like the palpitations that he or she associates with anxiety or exercise.
- Extrasystoles are described as the heart 'jumping' or 'missing a beat'. It is not possible to distinguish between supraventricular and ventricular extrasystoles from a patient's description.
- A paroxysmal tachycardia begins suddenly and sometimes stops suddenly. The heart is often 'too fast to count'. Severe attacks are associated with dizziness, breathlessness, and chest pain.

Table 3.1 compares the symptoms associated with sinus tachycardia and a paroxysmal tachycardia, and shows how a diagnosis can be made from the history.

Dizziness and syncope

These symptoms may have a cardiovascular or a neurological cause. Remember that cerebral hypoxia, however caused, may lead to a seizure and that can make the differentiation between cardiac and neurological syncope very difficult. The cardiovascular causes are:

- Simple faint. These always occur while standing, often in a hot or crowded room. Sinus bradycardia may make the pulse difficult to feel.
- Postural hypotension, occurring immediately on standing. It is seen in people with loss of blood volume, those with autonomic

Table 3.1 Diagnosis of sinus tachycardia or paroxysmal tachycardia from a patient's symptoms

Symptoms	Sinus tachycardia	Paroxysmal tachycardia
Timing of initial attack	Attacks probably began recently	Attacks probably began in teens or early adult life
Associations of attack	Exercise, anxiety	Usually no associations, but occasionally exercise-induced
Rate of start of palpitations	Slow build-up	Sudden onset
Rate of end of palpitations	'Die away'	Classically sudden, but often 'die away'
Heart rate	< 140/min	> 160/min
Associated symptoms	Paraesthesia due to hyperventilation	Chest pain, breathlessness, dizziness, syncope
Ways of terminating attacks	Relaxation	Breath holding, Valsalva's manoeuvre

nervous system disease (e.g. diabetes, Shy–Drager syndrome) and those who are being treated with anti-hypertensive drugs.

- Obstruction to blood flow in the heart or lungs, due to aortic stenosis, pulmonary embolus, pulmonary hypertension, hypertrophic cardiomyopathy or atrial myxoma.
- Arrhythmias. Dizziness and syncope occur with tachycardias, but the patient is usually aware of a fast heartbeat before becoming dizzy. Slow heart rates are often not appreciated – the classical cause is a Stokes–Adams attack due to a very slow ventricular rate in patients with complete heart block. A Stokes–Adams attack can be recognized because the patient is initially pale but flushes red on recovery.

Table 3.2 Physical signs and arrhythmias

Pulse	Heart rate (beats/min)	Possible nature of arrhythmia
Regular	< 50	Nodal escape rhythm
		Second or third degree block
	60–120	Probable sinus rhythm
	150	Probable atrial flutter with 2:1 block
	140–170	Nodal tachycardia
		Ventricular tachycardia
	> 180	Probable ventricular tachycardia
	300	Atrial flutter with 1:1 conduction
Irregular		Extrasystoles
		Atrial fibrillation
Jugular venous pulse		More pulsations visible than the heart rate – second or third degree block
		Cannon waves – third degree block

PHYSICAL EXAMINATION

If the patient has symptoms at the time of examination, the physical signs shown in Table 3.2 may point towards the nature of an arrhythmia.

If the patient has no symptoms at the time of the examination, look for:

• Evidence of any heart disease that might cause an arrhythmia
• Evidence of non-cardiac disease that might cause an arrhythmia
• Evidence of cardiovascular disease that might cause syncope without an arrhythmia.

Table 3.3 lists some of the rhythms and conditions associated with syncope and Table 3.4 gives the rhythms and underlying disease associated with palpitations.

Table 3.3 Conditions associated with syncope

Cardiac rhythm	Underlying cause
Sinus rhythm	Neurological diseases, including epilepsy Vagal overactivity: • simple faint • carotid sinus hypersensitivity • acute myocardial infarction Postural hypotension: • blood loss • hypotensive drugs • Addison's disease • autonomic dysfunction Circulatory obstruction: • aortic or pulmonary stenosis • hypertrophic cardiomyopathy • pulmonary embolus • pulmonary hypertension • atrial myxoma Drugs: • beta-blockers
Atrial fibrillation with slow ventricular rate	Rheumatic heart disease Ischaemic heart disease Cardiomyopathies Drugs: • digoxin • beta-blockers • verapamil • amiodarone
'Sick sinus' rhythms	Congenital Familial Idiopathic Ischaemic heart disease Rheumatic heart disease Cardiomyopathy Amyloidosis Collagen diseases Myocarditis Drugs: • lithium

Table 3.3 Contd

Cardiac rhythm	Underlying cause
Second or third degree block	Idiopathic (fibrosis) Congenital Ischaemia Aortic valve calcification Surgery or trauma Tumours in the His bundle Drugs: • digoxin • beta-blockers

Table 3.4 Conditions associated with palpitations

Cardiac rhythm	Underlying cause
Extrasystoles	Normal heart Any cardiac disease Anaemia
Sinus tachycardia	Normal heart Anxiety Anaemia Acute blood loss Pregnancy Lung disease CO_2 retention Pulmonary embolus Phaeochromocytoma
Atrial fibrillation	Rheumatic heart disease Thyrotoxicosis Ischaemic heart disease Cardiomyopathy Alcoholism Apparently normal heart with 'lone atrial fibrillation'
Supraventricular tachycardia	Pre-excitation syndromes Apparently normal heart
Ventricular tachycardia	Acute myocardial infarction Ischaemic heart disease Cardiomyopathy (hypertrophic or dilated) Long QT syndrome Myocarditis Drugs Apparently normal heart: idiopathic

It is only possible to make a confident diagnosis that an arrhythmia is the cause of palpitations or syncope if an ECG recording of the arrhythmia can be obtained, and if it can be shown that the occurrence of the arrhythmia coincides with the patient's symptoms.

If the patient is asymptomatic at the time of examination it may be worth arranging for an ECG to be recorded during an attack of palpitations, or to be recorded continuously on a tape recorder (the 'Holter' technique) in the hope that an episode of the arrhythmia will be detected.

THE ECG WHEN THE PATIENT IS ASYMPTOMATIC

Even when the patient is asymptomatic, the resting ECG can be very helpful.

Syncope due to cardiac disease other than arrhythmias
The ECG may indicate that syncopal attacks have a cardiovascular cause other than an arrhythmia.

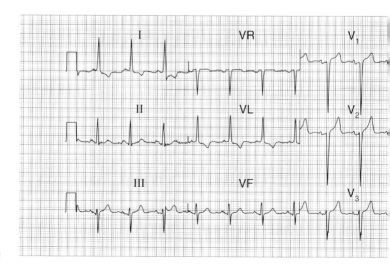

ECG evidence of left ventricular hypertrophy or of left bundle branch block (LBBB) may suggest that syncope is due to aortic stenosis. The ECGs in Figures 3.1 and 3.2 were recorded from patients who had syncopal attacks on exercise due to severe aortic stenosis

ECG evidence of right ventricular hypertrophy suggests thromboembolic pulmonary hypertension. The ECG in Figure 3.3 is that of a middle-aged woman with dizziness on exertion, due to multiple pulmonary emboli.

Syncope due to hypertrophic cardiomyopathy may be associated with a characteristic ECG that resembles that of patients with anterior ischaemia (Fig. 3.4) (see Ch. 4). In each case, the patient and the ECG must be judged together to arrive at a diagnosis. Hypertrophic cardiomyopathy can cause syncope due to obstruction to outflow from the left ventricle, or can cause symptomatic arrhythmias.

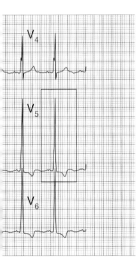

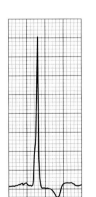

Fig. 3.1 Left ventricular hypertrophy

Note
- Sinus rhythm
- Bifid P waves suggest left atrial hypertrophy (best seen in lead V_4)
- Normal axis
- Tall R waves and deep S waves
- T waves inverted in leads I, VL, V_5, V_6

Tall R wave, inverted T wave in lead V_5

117

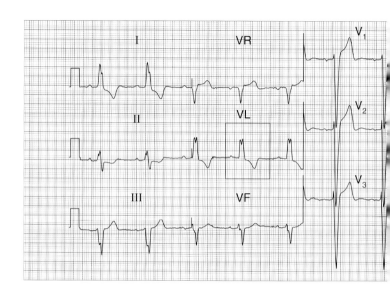

Fig. 3.3 **Right ventricular hypertrophy**

Note
- Sinus rhythm
- Right axis deviation
- Dominant R waves in lead V_1
- Inverted T waves in leads V_1–V_4

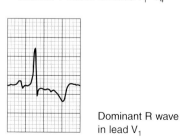

Dominant R wave
in lead V_1

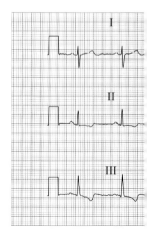

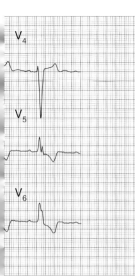

Fig. 3.2 Left bundle branch block

Note
- Sinus rhythm
- Slight PR interval prolongation (212 ms)
- Broad QRS complexes
- 'M' pattern in lateral leads
- T wave inversion in leads I, VL, V_5, V_6

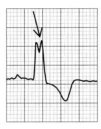

M pattern of LBBB in lead VL

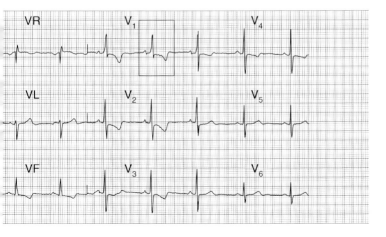

119

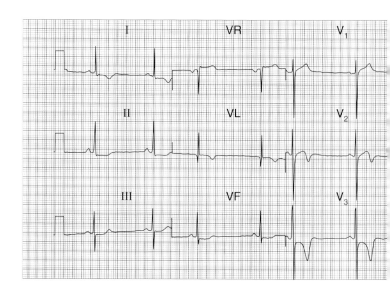

Patients with possible tachycardias

Mitral stenosis

Mitral stenosis leads to atrial fibrillation, but when the heart is still in sinus rhythm the presence of the characteristics of left atrial hypertrophy on the ECG may give a clue that paroxysmal atrial fibrillation is occurring (Fig. 3.5).

Pre-excitation syndromes

In the pre-excitation syndromes, abnormal pathways connect the atria and ventricles, forming an anatomical basis for re-entry tachycardia (see Ch. 1).

In the Wolff–Parkinson–White (WPW) syndrome, an accessory pathway connects either the left atrium and left ventricle, or the right atrium and right ventricle. In either case the normal atrioventricular (AV) nodal delay is bypassed, so the PR interval is short. Ventricular activation is initially abnormal, causing a slurred upstroke of the R wave, but later activation spreading normally through the AV node and His bundle is normal.

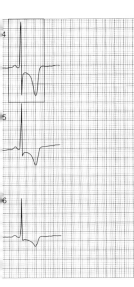

Fig. 3.4 Hypertrophic cardiomyopathy

Note
- Sinus rhythm
- Marked T wave inversion in leads V_3–V_6

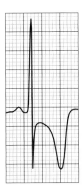

Inverted T wave in lead V_4

With a left-sided accessory pathway, the ECG shows a dominant R wave in lead V_1. This is called a 'type A' pattern (Fig. 3.6). This pattern of WPW conduction can easily be mistaken for right ventricular hypertrophy, the differentiation being made by the presence or absence of a short PR interval.

The ECG in Figure 3.7 is from a young man who complained of symptoms that sounded like paroxysmal tachycardia. His ECG shows WPW syndrome type A, but it would be quite easy to miss the short PR interval unless the whole of the 12-lead trace were carefully inspected. The short PR interval and delta waves are most obvious in leads V_4 and V_5.

When the accessory pathway is on the right side of the heart, there is no dominant R wave in lead V_1 and this is called a 'type B' pattern (Fig. 3.8).

ECGs indicating pre-excitation of the WPW type are found in approximately 1 in every 3000 healthy young people. Only half of these ever have an episode of tachycardia, and many have only very occasional attacks.

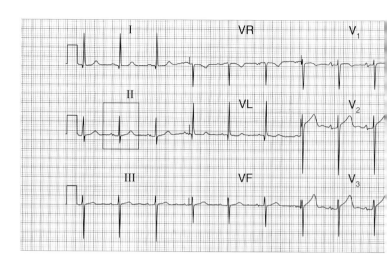

Fig. 3.6 Wolff–Parkinson–White syndrome, type A

Note
- Sinus rhythm
- Short PR interval
- Broad QRS complexes
- Slurred upstroke to QRS complexes – the delta wave
- Inverted T waves in leads II,III,VF, V_1–V_4

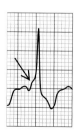

Delta wave in lead III

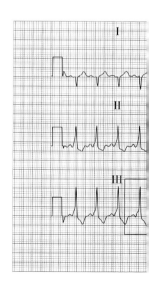

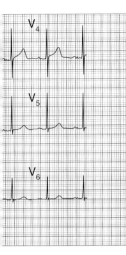

Fig. 3.5 Left atrial hypertrophy

Note
- Sinus rhythm
- Bifid P waves most clearly seen in leads I, II, V_3–V_5

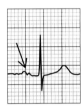

Bifid P wave in lead II

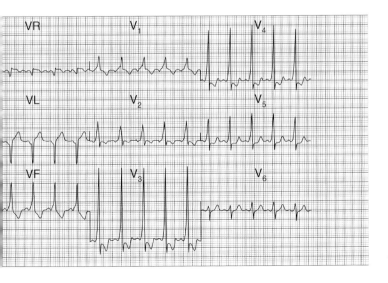

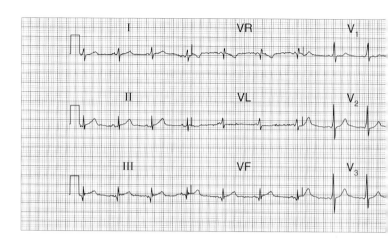

Fig. 3.8 Wolff–Parkinson–White syndrome, type B

Note
- Sinus rhythm
- Short PR interval
- Broad QRS complexes with delta waves
- No dominant R waves in lead V$_1$ (cf. Figs 3.6 and 3.7)
- T wave inversion in leads III, VF, V$_3$

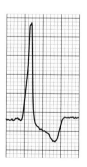

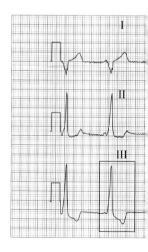

Short PR interval, broad QRS complex, in lead III

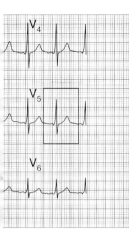

Fig. 3.7 Wolff–Parkinson–White syndrome, type A

Note

- Sinus rhythm
- Short PR interval, especially obvious in leads V_3–V_5
- Slurred upstroke to QRS complexes obvious in leads V_3–V_5 but not obvious in the limb leads
- No T wave inversion in the anterior leads (cf. Fig. 3.6)

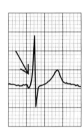

Delta wave in lead V_5

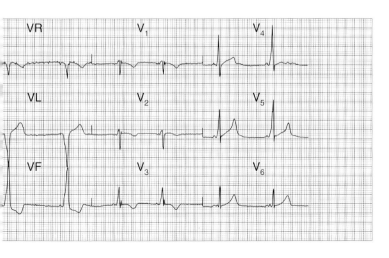

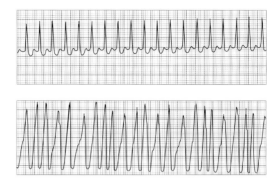

Fig. 3.9 Tachycardias in Wolff–Parkinson–White syndrome

Note
- The upper trace shows a narrow complex (orthodromic) tachycardia
- The lower trace shows a wide complex (antidromic) tachycardia
- In the lower trace the marked irregularity and variation of the complexes suggest that the rhythm is atrial fibrillation
- The underlying diagnosis of WPW syndrome is not apparent from either trace

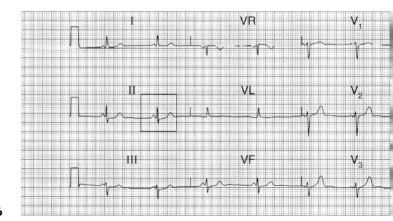

The physiological mechanisms involved in the tachycardias of the WPW syndrome are discussed in Chapter 1. During an episode of re-entry tachycardia, the QRS complex is usually narrow and the pattern resembles a junctional tachycardia – the presence of a pre-excitation syndrome may not be suspected.

The broad complex tachycardias which occur in patients with the WPW syndrome may resemble ventricular tachycardia. In most cases, the underlying rhythm is probably atrial fibrillation with anomalous atrioventricular conduction. This is a serious arrhythmia because ventricular fibrillation may occur (Fig. 3.9).

Where a bypass connects the atria to the bundle of His rather than to the right or left ventricle, there will be a short PR interval but the QRS complex will be normal. This is called the Lown–Ganong–Levine (LGL) syndrome (Fig. 3.10).

The short and fixed PR interval of pre-excitation must be distinguished from the short and varying PR interval of an accelerated idionodal rhythm ('wandering pacemaker'), shown in Figure 3.11. This ECG was recorded from an asymptomatic athlete.

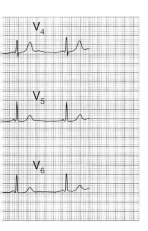

Fig. 3.10 Lown–Ganong–Levine syndrome

Note
- Sinus rhythm
- Short PR interval
- Normal QRS complexes and P waves

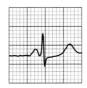

Short PR interval in lead II

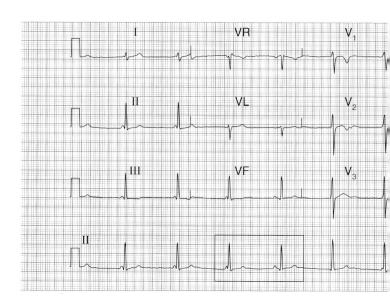

The long QT syndrome

Delayed repolarization occurs for a variety of reasons and causes a long QT interval. A prolonged QT interval is associated with paroxysmal ventricular tachycardia and therefore can be the cause of episodes of collapse or even of sudden death. Some causes of a prolonged QT interval are:

- Congenital
  - Jervell–Lange–Nielson syndrome
  - Romano–Ward syndrome
- Antiarrhythmic drugs
  - quinidine
  - procainamide
  - disopyramide
  - amiodarone
  - sotalol
- Other drugs
  - ketanserin

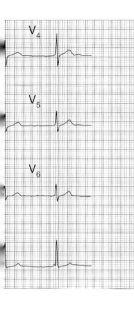

Fig. 3.11 Accelerated idionodal rhythm

Note
- Sinus rhythm
- Sinus rate is constant
- QRS rate is slightly faster than the sinus rate
- Variation of PR interval
- Normal QRS complexes

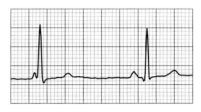

Variation of PR interval

- – tricyclic antidepressants
- – erythromycin
- – thioridazine
- Plasma electrolyte abnormality
  - – low potassium
  - – low magnesium
  - – low calcium.

The ECG in Figure 3.12 is from a 10-year-old girl who suffered from 'fainting' attacks. Her sister had died suddenly; three other siblings and both parents had normal ECGs.

The ECG in Figure 3.13 is from a patient who had a posterior myocardial infarction (see Ch. 4). He was treated with amiodarone because of recurrent ventricular tachycardias, and developed a prolonged QT interval. Figure 3.14 shows his record 4 months later: the prolonged QT interval reverted to normal when the amiodarone treatment was stopped.

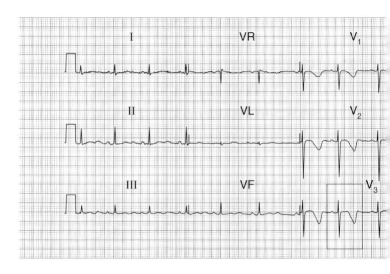

Fig. 3.13 Prolonged QT interval due to amiodarone

Note
- Sinus rhythm
- Normal axis
- Dominant R waves in lead V_1 due to posterior infarction
- QT interval 652 ms
- Bizarre T wave shape in anterior leads

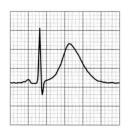

Long QT interval and bizarre T wave in lead V_2

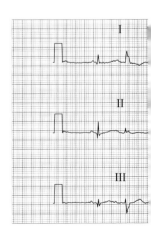

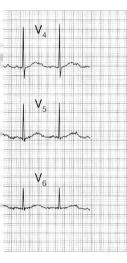

Fig. 3.12 Congenital long QT syndrome

Note
- Sinus rhythm
- Normal axis
- QT interval 520 ms
- Marked T wave inversion in leads V_2–V_4

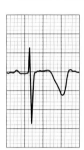

Long QT interval and inverted T wave in lead V_3

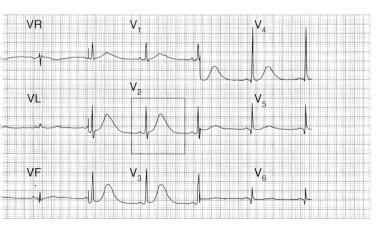

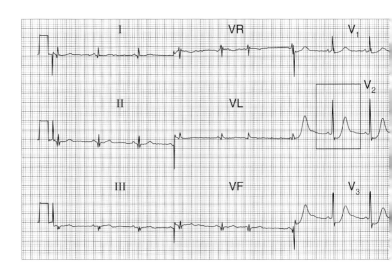

When a prolonged QT interval is associated with ventricular tachycardia, this usually involves a continuous change from upright to downward QRS complexes. This is called 'torsade de pointes'. The congenital long QT syndrome causes episodes of loss of consciousness at times of increased sympathetic nervous system activity. Such episodes occur in about 8% of affected subjects each year, and the annual death rate due to arrhythmias is about 1% of patients with a long QT syndrome. The ECG in Figure 3.15 was recorded from a young girl with a congenital long QT syndrome.

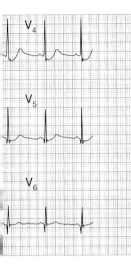

Fig. 3.14 Posterior infarct with normal QT interval

Note
- Same patient as in Figure 3.13
- Sinus rhythm
- Normal axis
- Dominant R waves in lead V_1
- Ischaemic ST segment depression
- Normal QT interval

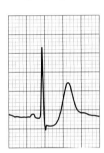

ST segment depression in lead V_2

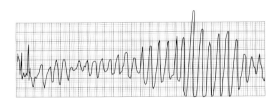

Fig. 3.15 Torsade de pointes

Note
- Broad complex tachycardia at 300/min
- Continually changing shape of QRS complexes

133

The Brugada syndrome
Sudden collapse due to ventricular tachycardia and fibrillation
occurs in a congenital disorder of sodium ion transport called
the Brugada syndrome. Between attacks, the ECG superficially
resembles that associated with RBBB, with an RSR[1] pattern in
leads V_1 and V_2 (Fig. 3.16). However, the ST segment in these leads
is raised, and there is no wide S wave in V_6 as there is in RBBB.
The changes are seen in the right ventricular leads because the
abnormal sodium channels are predominantly found in the right
ventricle. The ECG abnormality can be transient – the ECG in
Figure 3.17 was taken a day later from the same patient.

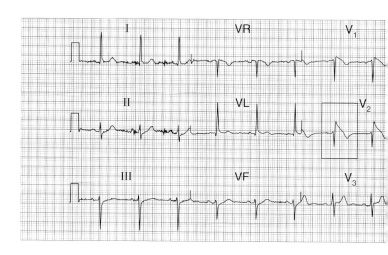

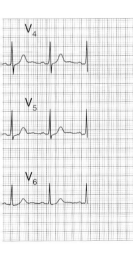

Fig. 3.16 Brugada syndrome

Note
- Sinus rhythm
- Normal axis
- Normal QRS complex duration
- RSR^1 pattern on leads V$_1$, V$_2$
- No wide S wave in lead V$_6$
- Raised, downward-sloping ST segment in leads V$_1$, V$_2$

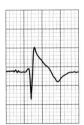

RSR^1 pattern and raised ST segment in lead V$_2$

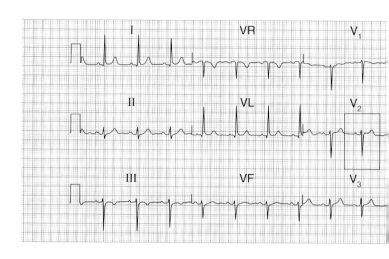

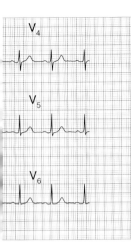

Fig. 3.17 Brugada syndrome

Note
• Same patient as in Figure 3.16
• Normal ECG

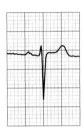

Normal appearance in
lead V_2

Patients with possible bradycardias

When a patient is asymptomatic, an intermittent bradycardia
can be suspected if the ECG shows any evidence of a conduction
defect. Nevertheless, it must be remembered that conduction
defects are quite common in healthy people and their presence
may be coincidental.

In a patient with syncopal attacks, ECG changes that would
be ignored in a healthy person take on a greater significance. First
and second degree block, themselves of no clinical importance,
may point to intermittent complete block. The ECGs in Figures
3.18, 3.19 and 3.20 are from patients with syncopal attacks, all of
whom eventually needed permanent pacemakers.

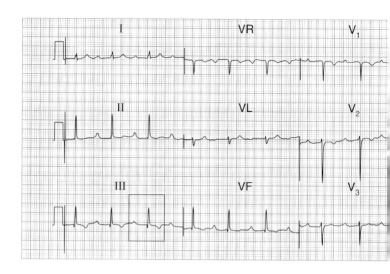

Fig. 3.19 Second degree block (Wenckebach)

Note

- Sinus rhythm
- PR interval lengthens progressively from 360 ms to 440 ms and then a P wave is not conducted
- Small Q wave and inverted T wave in leads III, VF suggest an old inferior infarct

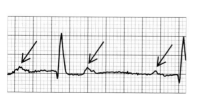

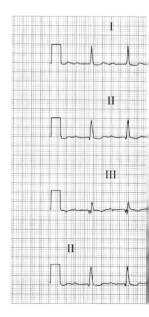

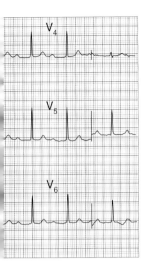

Fig. 3.18 First degree block

Note
- Sinus rhythm
- PR interval 380 ms
- T wave inversion in leads III, VF suggests ischaemia

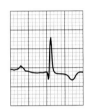

Long PR interval in lead III

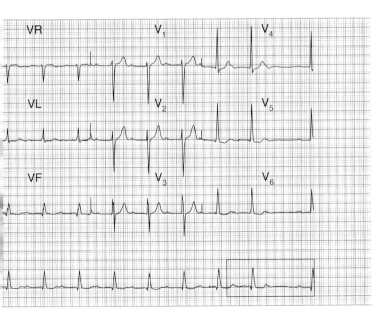

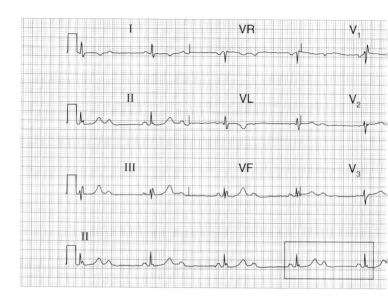

Combinations of conduction abnormalities

Left axis deviation usually indicates left anterior hemiblock, and when the QRS complex is narrow it can be accepted as a normal variant (Fig. 3.21).

A widened QRS complex with marked left axis deviation represents the full pattern of left anterior hemiblock (Fig. 3.22).

When left anterior hemiblock is associated with first degree block and LBBB (Fig. 3.23), both fascicles of the left bundle fail to conduct and conduction is also delayed in either the AV node, the His bundle or the right bundle branch.

Alternatively, the combination of first degree block and RBBB (Fig. 3.24) shows that conduction has failed in the right bundle branch and is also beginning to fail elsewhere.

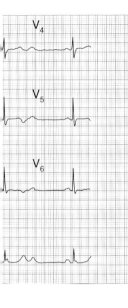

Fig. 3.20 Second degree block (2:1)

Note
- Sinus rhythm
- Alternate beats conducted and not conducted
- Lateral T wave inversion in leads I, VL, V$_6$ suggests ischaemia

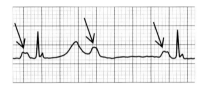

P waves

The combination of left anterior hemiblock and RBBB means that conduction into the ventricles is only passing through the posterior fascicle of the left bundle branch (Fig. 3.25). This is called 'bifascicular block'.

The combination of left anterior hemiblock, RBBB and first degree block suggests that there is disease in the remaining conducting pathway – either in the main His bundle or in the posterior fascicle of the left bundle branch. This is sometimes called 'trifascicular block' (Fig. 3.26). Complete conduction block in the right bundle and in both fascicles of the left bundle would, of course, cause complete (third degree) heart block.

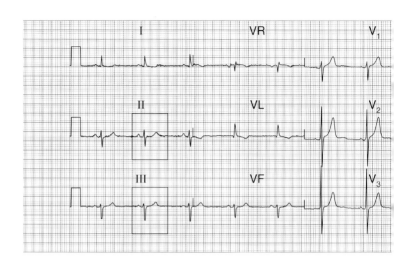

Fig. 3.22 Left anterior hemiblock

Note

- Sinus rhythm
- Left axis deviation
- Broad QRS complexes (122 ms)
- Inverted T waves in lead VL

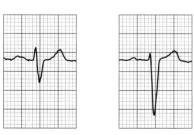

Dominant S waves and broad QRS complexes in leads II and III

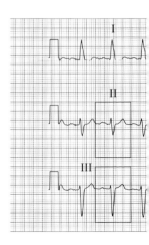

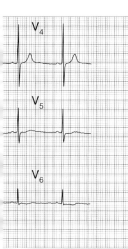

Fig. 3.21 Left axis deviation

Note
- Sinus rhythm
- Dominant S waves in leads II, III: left axis deviation
- Normal QRS complex duration
- Lateral T wave inversion

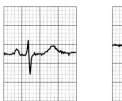 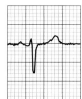

Dominant S waves in leads II and III

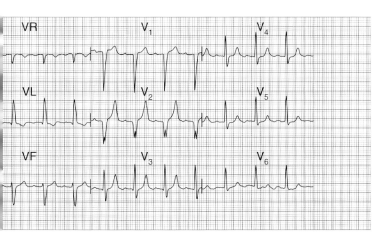

143

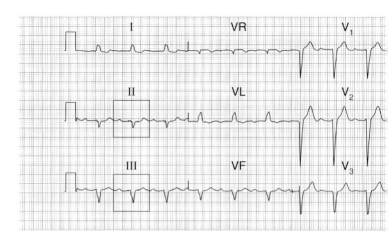

Fig. 3.24 **First degree block and right bundle branch block**

Note
- Sinus rhythm
- PR interval 328 ms
- Right axis deviation
- Broad QRS complexes
- RBBB pattern

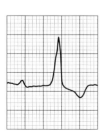

Long PR interval and RBBB pattern in lead V₁

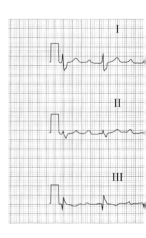

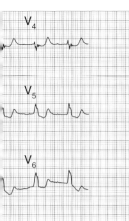

Fig. 3.23 First degree block and left anterior hemiblock

Note
- Sinus rhythm
- PR interval 300 ms
- Left anterior hemiblock
- Broad QRS complexes

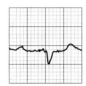 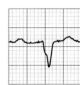

Long PR interval in leads II and III

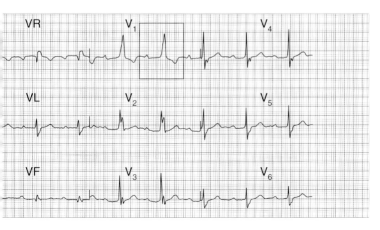

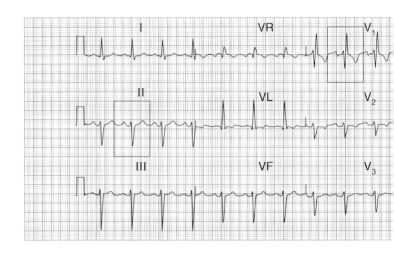

Fig. 3.26 Trifascicular block

Note
- Sinus rhythm
- PR interval 224 ms
- Left anterior hemiblock
- RBBB

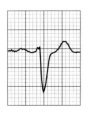

Left axis deviation
in lead II

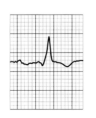

RBBB in lead V₁

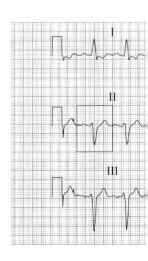

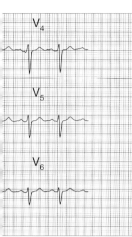

Fig. 3.25 Bifascicular block

Note
- Sinus rhythm
- PR interval normal (176 ms)
- Left anterior hemiblock
- RBBB

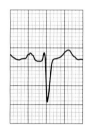

Left axis deviation and broad QRS complex in lead II

RBBB in lead V₁

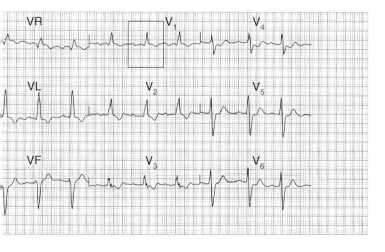

Right axis deviation is not necessarily a feature of left posterior hemiblock, but when combined with other evidence of conducting tissue disease such as first degree block (Fig. 3.27), it probably is.

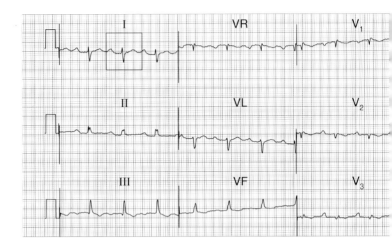

Fig. 3.28 Second degree block and left anterior hemiblock

Note
- Sinus rhythm
- Second degree block (2:1 type)
- Left anterior hemiblock
- Poor R wave progression suggests possible old anterior infarct

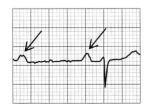

P waves in lead II

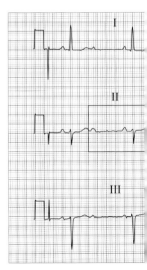

The combination of second degree (2:1) block with left anterior hemiblock (Fig. 3.28) or with both left anterior hemiblock and RBBB (Fig. 3.29) suggests widespread conduction tissue disease.

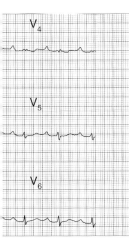

Fig. 3.27 Left posterior hemiblock

Note
- Sinus rhythm
- First degree block (PR interval 320 ms)
- Right axis deviation
- This could represent right ventricular hypertrophy, but there is no dominant R wave in lead V₁

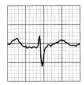

Long PR interval and deep S wave in lead I

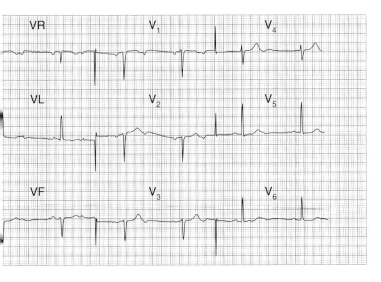

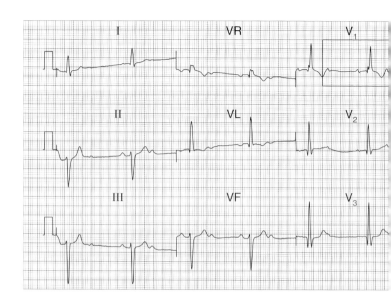

THE ECG WHEN THE PATIENT HAS SYMPTOMS

If an ECG can be recorded at the time when the patient has symptoms, then there can be little doubt about the relationship between the symptoms and the cardiac rhythm. Table 3.5 lists some of the things to look for and think about.

Table 3.5 ECG features between attacks of palpitations or syncope

ECG appearance	Possible cause of symptoms
ECG completely normal	Symptoms may not be due to a primary arrhythmia – consider anxiety, epilepsy, atrial myxoma or carotid sinus hypersensitivity

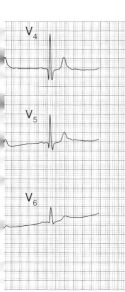

Fig. 3.29 Second degree block, left anterior hemiblock and right bundle branch block

Note
- Sinus rhythm
- Second degree block (2:1 type)
- Left anterior hemiblock
- RBBB

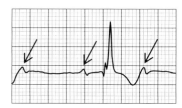

P waves and RBBB in lead V$_1$

Table 3.5 Contd

ECG appearance	Possible cause of symptoms
ECGs that suggest cardiac disease	Left ventricular hypertrophy or left bundle branch block: aortic stenosis Right ventricular hypertrophy: pulmonary hypertension Anterior T wave inversion: hypertrophic cardiomyopathy
ECGs that suggest intermittent tachyarrhythmia	Left atrial hypertrophy: mitral stenosis, so possibly atrial fibrillation Pre-excitation syndromes Long QT syndrome Flat T waves suggest hypokalaemia Digoxin effect: ?digoxin toxicity
ECGs that suggest intermittent bradyarrhythmia	Second degree block First degree block plus bundle branch block Digoxin effect

Sinus rhythm in patients with symptoms

Sinus rhythm can be irregular (sinus arrhythmia) but the patient is never aware of this. The ECG of a patient with sinus arrhythmia (Fig. 3.30) may suggest atrial extrasystoles – but in sinus rhythm, P wave morphology is constant while with atrial extrasystoles it varies.

Patients often complain of palpitations that are due to sinus tachycardia: the main causes are exercise, anxiety, thyrotoxicosis and the treatment of asthma with beta-adrenergic agonists. The ECG in Figure 3.31 shows sinus tachycardia from an unusual cause – the habitual drinking of large quantities of Coca-Cola.

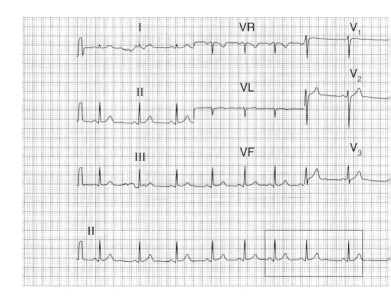

When sinus tachycardia results from anxiety, heart rates of up to 150/min are possible and the rhythm may be mistaken for an atrial tachycardia. Pressure on the carotid sinus will cause transient slowing of the heart rate and the P waves will become more obvious.

Marked sinus bradycardia is characteristic of athletic training, but is also part of the cause of symptoms in fainting (the 'vasovagal' attack). It may also contribute to hypotension and heart failure in patients with an inferior myocardial infarction.

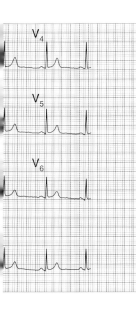

Fig. 3.30 Sinus arrhythmia

Note
- Sinus rhythm
- All P waves identical
- Progressive shortening then lengthening of the R–R interval

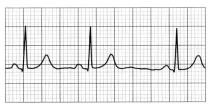

Identical P waves and irregular R–R interval

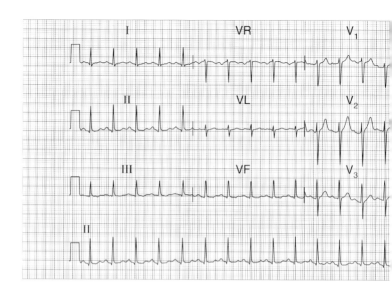

Extrasystoles in patients with symptoms

An ECG is necessary to differentiate between supraventricular and ventricular extrasystoles.

When extrasystoles have a supraventricular origin (Fig. 3.32), the QRS complex is narrow and both it and the T wave have the same configuration as in the sinus beat. Atrial extrasystoles have abnormal P waves. Junctional extrasystoles either have a P wave very close to the QRS complex (in front of it or behind it) or have no visible P waves.

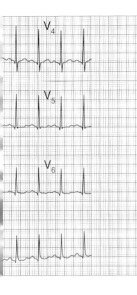

Fig. 3.31 Sinus tachycardia

Note
- Sinus rhythm at the rate of 120/min
- Nonspecific ST segment changes in leads III, VF, V$_6$

Ventricular extrasystoles produce wide QRS complexes of abnormal shape, and the T wave is also usually abnormal. No P waves are present (Fig. 3.33).

When a ventricular extrasystole appears on the upstroke of the preceding beat, the 'R on T' phenomenon is said to be present (Fig. 3.34). This can initiate ventricular fibrillation, but usually it does not do so.

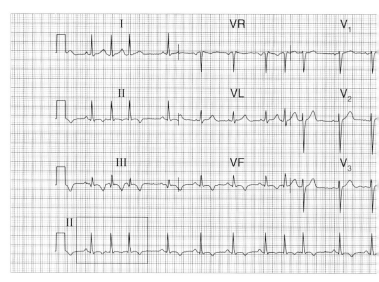

Fig. 3.33 Ventricular extrasystoles

Note

- Sinus rhythm with coupled ventricular extrasystoles
- Sinus beats show tall R waves and inverted T waves in leads V_5, V_6 (indicating left ventricular hypertrophy)
- Extrasystoles are of RBBB configuration, and their T wave inversion has no other significance

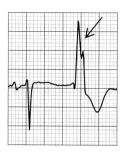

Extrasystole with RBBB configuration in lead V_1

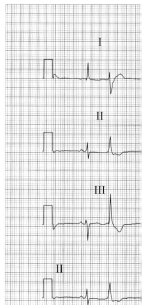

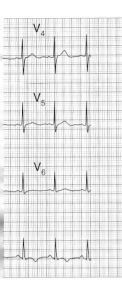

Fig. 3.32 Supraventricular extrasystoles

Note
- Sinus rhythm with atrial and junctional extrasystoles
- Normal axis
- Normal QRS complexes
- Inverted T waves in leads III, VF

First beat: normal; second beat: atrial extrasystole, with abnormal P wave; third beat: AV nodal (junctional) extrasystole, with no P wave

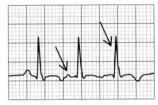

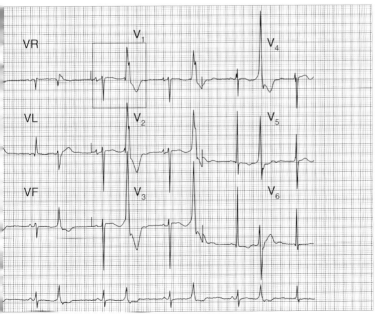

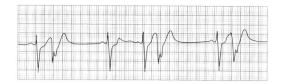

Fig. 3.34 R on T phenomenon

Note
- Ventricular extrasystoles occurring near the peak of the preceding T wave

Narrow complex tachycardias in patients with symptoms

The pathophysiology of the tachycardias is discussed in Chapter 1. This section concerns their diagnosis and management.

A tachycardia can be described as 'narrow complex' if the QRS

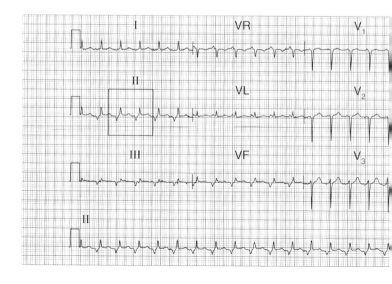

complex is of normal duration, i.e. < 120 ms. Properly speaking, sinus, atrial and junctional arrhythmias are all supraventricular, but the term 'supraventricular tachycardia' is often inappropriately used interchangeably with 'junctional tachycardia'. All these supraventricular rhythms have QRS complexes of normal shape and width, and the T waves have the same shape as in the sinus beat.

Atrial tachycardia
In atrial tachycardia (Fig. 3.35), P waves are present but they have an abnormal shape. They are sometimes hidden in the T wave of the preceding beat.

In atrial tachycardia the P wave rate is in the range 130–250/min. When the atrial rate exceeds about 180/min, physiological block will occur in the AV node, so that the ventricular rate becomes half that of the atria. Atrial tachycardia with 2:1 block is characteristic of (but not commonly seen with) digoxin toxicity.

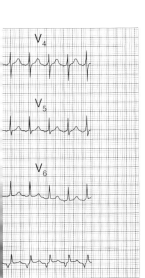

Fig. 3.35 Atrial tachycardia

Note
- Narrow complex tachycardia, heart rate 140/min
- Abnormal shaped P waves, one per QRS complex
- Short PR interval
- ECG otherwise normal

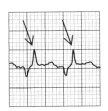

Abnormal P waves in lead II

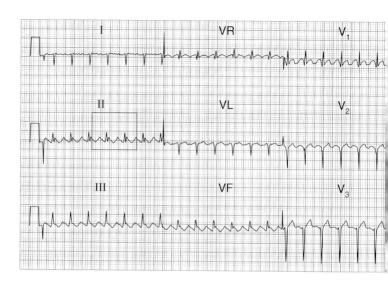

Atrial flutter

In atrial flutter, the atrial rate is 300/min and the P waves form a continuous 'sawtooth' line. As the AV node usually fails to conduct all the P waves, the relationship between P waves and QRS complexes is usually 2:1, 3:1, or 4:1. Figure 3.36 shows atrial flutter with 2:1 block, giving a ventricular rate of 150/min. The ECG in Figure 3.37 is from the same patient after reversion to sinus rhythm.

The ECC in Figure 3.38 shows atrial flutter with 4:1 block.

The ECG in Figure 3.39 shows a narrow complex (therefore supraventricular) rhythm with a rate of 300/min. In atrial flutter the atrial rate is 300/min therefore this is almost certainly atrial flutter with 1:1 conduction.

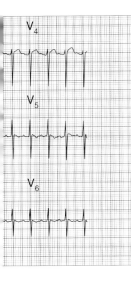

Fig. 3.36 Atrial flutter with 2:1 block

Note
- Regular narrow complex tachycardia
- 'Sawtooth' of atrial flutter most easily seen in lead II

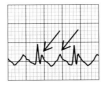

'Flutter' waves in lead II

If the ventricular rate is rapid and P waves cannot be seen, carotid sinus pressure will usually increase the block in the AV node and make the 'sawtooth' more obvious (see p. 227).

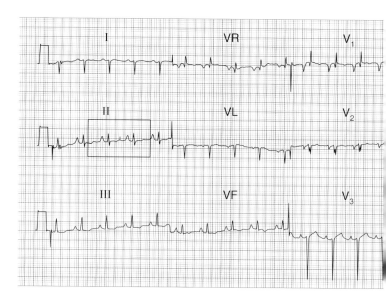

Fig. 3.38 Atrial flutter with 4:1 block

Note
- With 4:1 block and a ventricular rate of 72/min, flutter waves can be seen in all leads

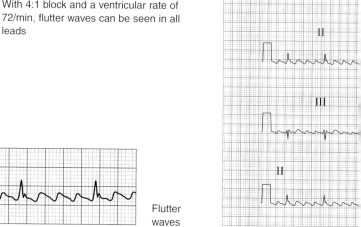

Flutter waves

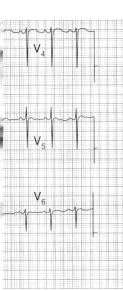

Fig. 3.37 Sinus rhythm, post-cardioversion

Note
- Same patient as in Figure 3.36
- Sinus rhythm
- Right axis deviation
- Dominant R waves in lead V_1
- Deep S waves in lead V_6, suggesting right ventricular hypertrophy
- The cardiac axis and QRS complexes have not been changed by cardioversion

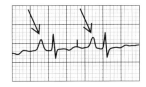

P waves in
lead II

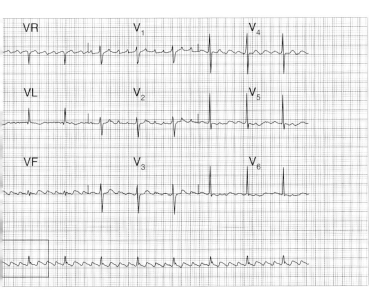

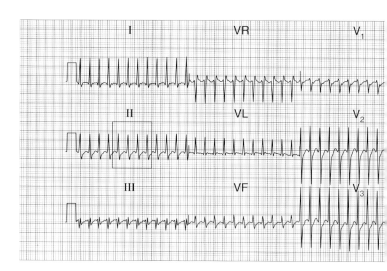

Junctional or atrioventricular re-entry tachycardia
Junctional tachycardia is caused by re-entry of the electrical
impulse via a double conducting channel within, or very close to,
the AV node (see Ch. 1). Junctional tachycardia is therefore now
usually called 'atrioventricular re-entry' (AVRE) tachycardia. In
this rhythm no P waves can be seen. Carotid sinus pressure either
reverts the heart to sinus rhythm or has no effect.

The ECG in Figure 3.40 shows a narrow complex tachycardia
at 150/min, without any obvious P waves. After reversion to sinus
rhythm (Fig. 3.41) the shape of the QRS complexes does not
change.

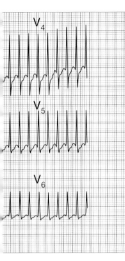

Fig. 3.39 Atrial flutter with 1:1 conduction

Note
- Narrow complex tachycardia at nearly 300/min
- No P waves visible
- Ventricular rate suggests that the underlying rhythm is atrial flutter

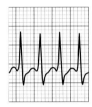

Narrow complex tachycardia at 300/min in lead II

The ECG in Figure 3.42 shows what appears to be a straightforward AV nodal re-entry tachycardia, but on return to sinus rhythm (Fig. 3.43) it shows a WPW pattern. The tachycardia was therefore orthodromic, with the re-entry circuit involving anterograde (normal) conduction down the AV node and His bundle (see Ch. 1).

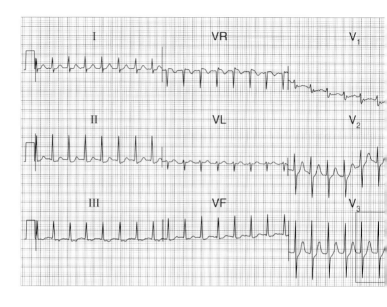

Fig. 3.41 Sinus rhythm following cardioversion

Note
- Sinus rhythm
- QRS complexes and T waves are the same shape as in AVRE tachycardia (Fig. 3.40)
- Now no suggestion of ischaemia

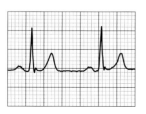

Sinus rhythm in lead II

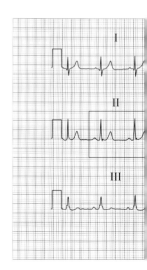

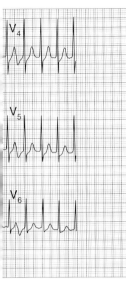

Fig. 3.40 Atrioventricular re-entry tachycardia

Note
- Regular narrow complex tachycardia, rate 150/min
- No P waves visible
- ST segment depression in leads II, III, VF suggests ischaemia

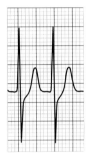

Narrow complexes at 150/min in lead V₃

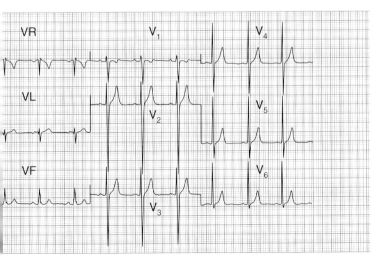

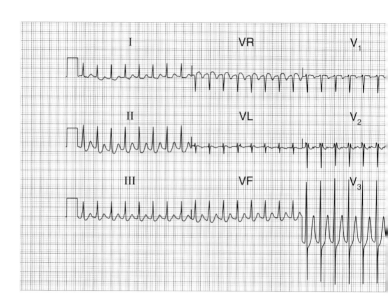

Fig. 3.43 Sinus rhythm, WPW syndrome

Note

- Same patient as in Figure 3.42
- Sinus rhythm
- Short PR interval
- Broad QRS complexes with delta wave
- Dominant R wave in lead V_1 shows WPW syndrome type A

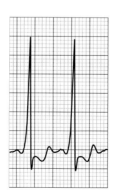

Short PR interval and delta wave in lead V_4

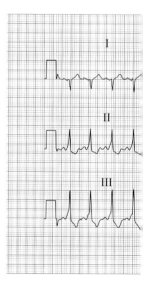

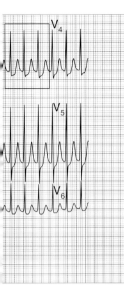

Fig. 3.42 Supraventricular tachycardia

Note
- Narrow complex tachycardia
- No P waves visible
- Some ST segment depression, suggesting ischaemia

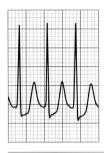

Narrow complexes with ST segment depression in lead V₄

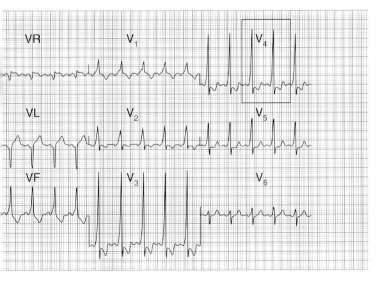

Atrial fibrillation

In atrial fibrillation, disorganized atrial activity causes the P waves to disappear and the ECG baseline becomes totally irregular (Fig. 3.44). At times atrial activity may become sufficiently synchronized for a 'flutter-like' pattern to appear, but this rapidly breaks up (Fig. 3.45). In atrial fibrillation, as opposed to atrial flutter, the QRS complexes are totally irregular.

Broad complex tachycardias in patients with symptoms

'Broad complex' tachycardias are those in which the QRS complex duration exceeds 120 ms and which are not due to sinus rhythm with bundle branch block. Broad complexes can be the result of a supraventricular tachycardia with bundle branch block, or of ventricular tachycardia (VT). A supraventricular origin for a broad

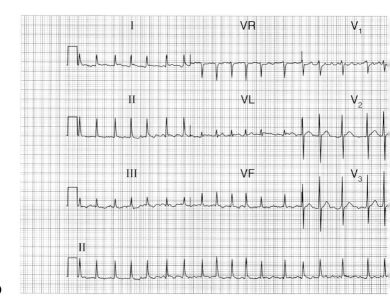

complex tachycardia can only be diagnosed with certainty when there is intermittent sinus rhythm with the same QRS complex configuration as is seen in the tachycardia (Fig. 3.46).

Here we are concerned with broad complex rhythms without obvious P waves. These could be atrial fibrillation or junctional rhythms with bundle branch block, or could be ventricular rhythms. The differentiation of these can be difficult. You cannot distinguish between supraventricular and ventricular rhythms by the clinical state of the patient. Either type of rhythm can be well tolerated, and either can lead to cardiovascular collapse. However, broad complex tachycardias occurring in thecourse of an acute myocardial infarction (which is when they are most often seen) are almost always ventricular in origin.

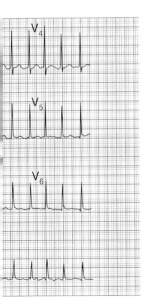

Fig. 3.44 Atrial fibrillation

Note
- Irregular narrow complex tachycardia at 150/min
- During long R–R intervals, irregular baseline can be seen
- Suggestion of flutter waves in lead V_1

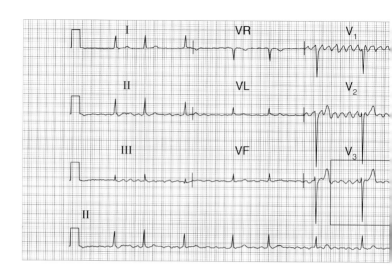

With these things in mind, the ECG should be analysed logically. Look in turn for the following features:

1. The presence of P waves. If there is one P wave per QRS complex, it must be sinus rhythm with bundle branch block. If P waves can be seen at a slower rate than the QRS complexes, it must be VT.
2. The QRS complex duration. If longer than 160 ms, it is probably VT.
3. QRS complex regularity. VT is usually regular.. An irregular broad complex tachycardia usually means atrial fibrillation with abnormal conduction.
4. The cardiac axis. VT is usually associated with left axis deviation.
5. QRS complex configuration. If the QRS complexes in the V leads all point either upwards or downwards ('concordance') it is probably VT.
6. When the QRS complex shows an RBBB pattern, abnormal conduction is more likely if the second R peak is higher than the first. VT is likely if the first R peak is higher.
7. The presence of fusion and capture beats indicates that the broad complexes are due to VT (see p. 190).

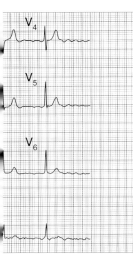

Fig. 4.45 Atrial fibrillation

Note
- Irregular narrow complex rhythm
- Apparent flutter waves in lead V_1, but these are not constant and from leads II and V_3 it is clear that this is atrial fibrillation

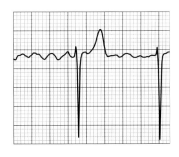

Atrial fibrillation in lead V_3

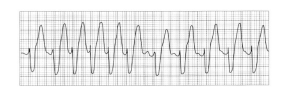

Fig. 3.46 Junctional tachycardia with bundle branch block

Note
- A single sinus beat with a broad QRS complex is followed by five beats without P waves, but with the same broad QRS pattern
- Sinus rhythm is then restored and the QRS complex remains unchanged
- The tachycardia must be supraventricular with bundle branch block

173

P waves

The ECG in Figure 3.47 is from a patient with an acute infarction, and shows a broad complex rhythm at about 110/min. One P wave per QRS complex can clearly be seen, and this is obviously sinus rhythm with LBBB.

The ECG in Figure 3.48 shows a very irregular broad complex rhythm with no obvious P waves. There is an obvious LBBB pattern in leads V_5 and V_6. Whether the R–R interval is short or long, the appearance of the QRS complex is the same. The irregularity is the key to the diagnosis of atrial fibrillation with LBBB.

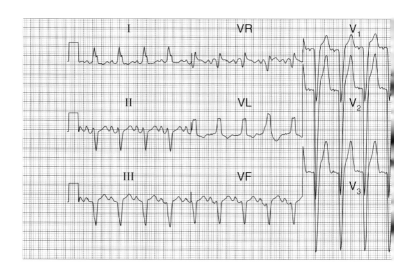

The ECG in Figure 3.49 is also an example of atrial fibrillation and LBBB, but this is not quite as obvious as in Figure 3.48. The QRS complexes at first sight may appear regular, but on close inspection they are not. The LBBB is also not so obvious, but can be seen in lead I.

Occasionally it may be possible to identify P waves with a slower rate than the QRS complexes, indicating that the QRS complexes must be ventricular in origin. A 12-lead ECG during the tachycardia is important, because P waves may be visible in some leads but not in others (Fig. 3.50).

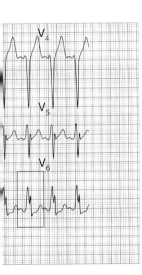

Fig. 3.47 Sinus rhythm with left bundle branch block

Note
- Sinus rhythm
- Left axis deviation
- Wide QRS complexes of LBBB configuration

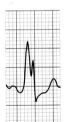

M wave of LBBB in lead V_6

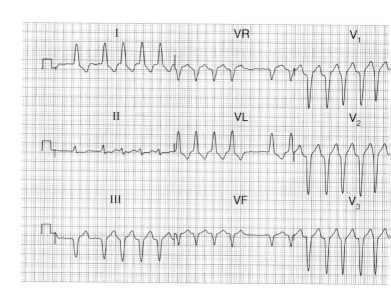

Fig. 3.49 Atrial fibrillation with left bundle branch block

Note

- Broad complex rhythm at 140/min
- Slightly irregular rhythm, best seen in lead V_6
- LBBB pattern, most obvious in lead I

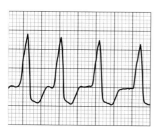

Irregular rhythm in lead V_6

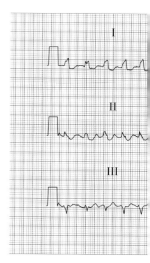

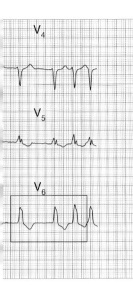

Fig. 3.48 Atrial fibrillation with left bundle branch block

Note
- Recorded at half sensitivity (0.5 cm = 1 mV)
- Irregular broad complex tachycardia
- No obvious P waves, but irregular baseline in lead VR
- LBBB configuration of QRS complexes

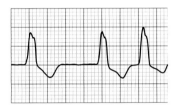

M wave of LBBB in lead V_6

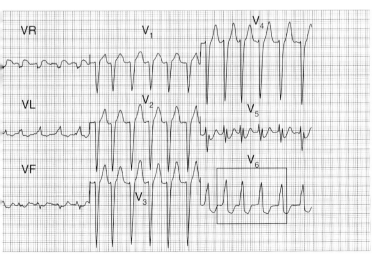

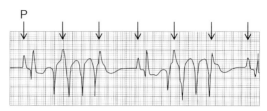

Fig. 3.50 Ventricular tachycardia

Note
- A single sinus beat is followed by a broad complex tachycardia
- During the tachycardia, P waves can still be seen at a normal rate (arrowed)
- So the broad complex tachycardia must have a ventricular origin

The QRS complex

The ECG in Figure 3.51 shows a broad complex tachycardia recorded from a patient with an acute infarction, and there is no question that this represents VT. The important features are:

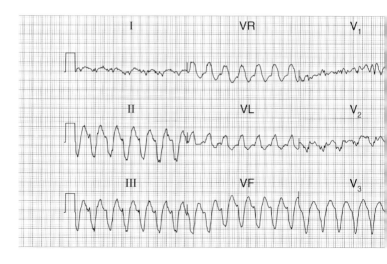

- Regular rhythm at 160/min (a fairly typical rate)
- Very broad complexes of 188 ms duration (when the QRS complex duration is > 160 ms, VT is likely)
- Left axis deviation
- In the V leads the QRS complexes all point in the same direction (in this case downwards). This is called 'concordance'.

The ECG in Figure 3.52 shows an ECG from another patient with an acute infarction. The shape of the QRS complexes is different from that in Figure 3.51, but the principles are the same:

- The rhythm is regular.
- The complexes are very broad.
- There is left axis deviation.
- The complexes show concordance.

The ECG in Figure 3.53 shows another example of VT, but this time the axis is normal. Unfortunately the 'rules' for diagnosing VT are not absolute and one or more of the features above may not be present.

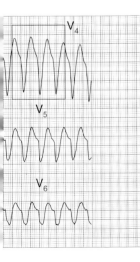

Fig. 3.51 Ventricular tachycardia

Note
- Regular broad complex tachycardia at 160/min
- Appearance of lead V_1 is clearly an artefact
- Left axis deviation
- All complexes point downwards (concordance)

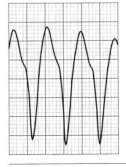

Broad complexes in lead V_4

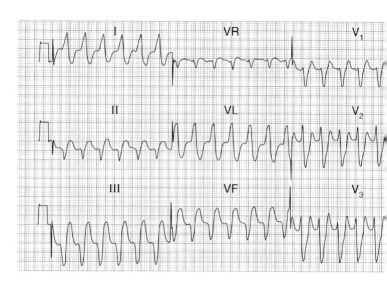

Fig. 3.53 Ventricular tachycardia

Note
- Regular broad complex tachycardia
- No P waves
- Normal axis
- Concordance (downward) of QRS complexes

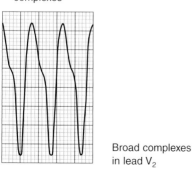

Broad complexes in lead V₂

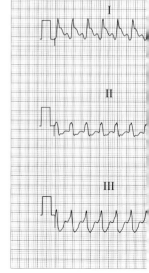

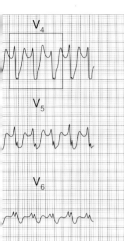

Fig. 3.52 Ventricular tachycardia

Note
- Regular broad complex tachycardia at 150/min
- No P waves visible
- Left axis deviation
- Concordance of QRS complexes in chest leads

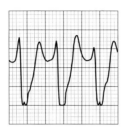

Broad complexes in lead V₄

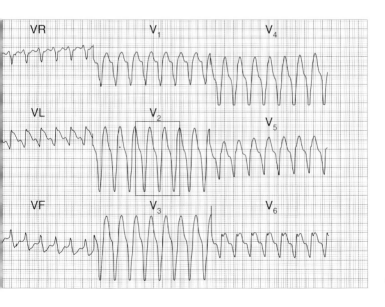

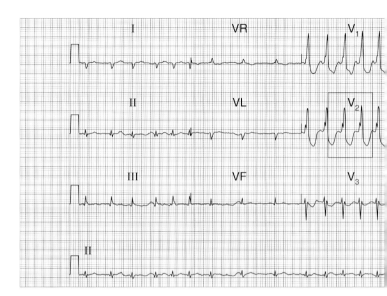

The ECG in Figure 3.54 shows atrial fibrillation with an abnormal QRS complex, the duration of which is just within the normal range of 116 ms. The RSR[1] pattern, most obviously seen in lead V_2, and the slurred S wave in lead V_6, show that this is 'partial RBBB'. Note that the second R peak of the QRS complex (the 'R[1]') is higher than first peak. This is characteristic of RBBB.

The ECG in Figure 3.55 shows a regular tachycardia with no P waves and a QRS complex showing a RBBB pattern. The duration of the QRS complex is at the upper limit of normal at 120 ms. This might be a supraventricular (probably junctional) tachycardia with RBBB conduction, or it may be a fascicular tachycardia. A fascicular tachycardia usually arises in the posterior fascicle of the left bundle branch. Typically there is left axis deviation (not present here). This is an unusual rhythm with a benign prognosis, and typically responds to verapamil.

The ECG in Figure 3.56 shows how difficult differentiation between supraventricular and ventricular rhythms can be. Some features suggest a supraventricular, and some a ventricular, origin of the rhythm.

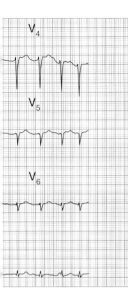

Fig. 3.54 Atrial fibrillation with right bundle branch block

Note

- Irregular broad complex tachycardia
- Right axis deviation
- QRS complexes shows RBBB pattern, with second R peak higher than the first

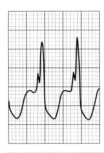

R^1 taller than R peak in lead V$_2$

Often only a comparison of the patient's ECGs taken when the tachycardia is present and when the patient is in sinus rhythm will establish the nature of the tachycardia. In any patient with a tachycardia it is essential to look through the old notes, to see if any ECGs have been recorded previously. The ECG in Figure 3.57 shows a broad complex tachycardia rather similar to that shown in Figure 3.56. This patient was in pain and was hypotensive, so he was cardioverted, and Figure 3.58 shows the post-cardioversion record.

Figure 3.59 shows the ECG from a patient admitted to hospital with an inferior myocardial infarction, who was initially in atrial fibrillation.

The patient then developed a broad complex tachycardia (Fig. 3.60). In the context of an acute infarction this would almost certainly be VT, and a comparison of Figure 3.60 with the ECG in atrial fibrillation (Fig. 3.59) shows the combination of left axis deviation and an RBBB. The change of axis is a strong pointer to a ventricular origin of the rhythm.

183

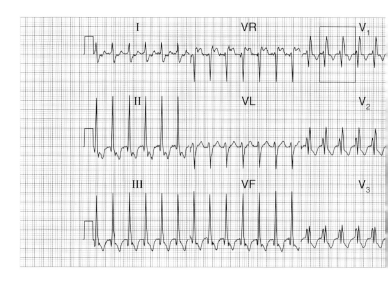

Fig. 3.56 Broad complex tachycardia, probably ventricular

Note

- Regular rhythm at 195/min
- Right axis deviation (suggests a supraventricular tachycardia with bundle branch block)
- Very broad complexes with QRS duration 200 ms (the primary evidence for VT)
- QRS complexes in lead V_1 points upwards, while complexes in V_6 point downwards: no concordance (suggests a supraventricular tachycardia)
- The second R peak (R^1) is greater than R peak in the QRS complexes in lead V_1 (suggests a supraventricular tachycardia)

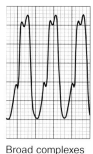

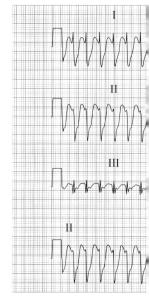

Broad complexes

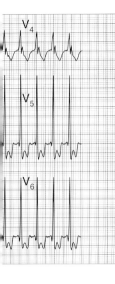

Fig. 3.55 ?Junctional tachycardia with right bundle branch block or ?fascicular tachycardia

Note

- Regular rhythm at 150/min
- Normal axis (R and S waves equal in lead I)
- QRS complex duration 120 ms (upper limit of normal)
- The second R peak (R^1) is taller than R peak in the QRS complex

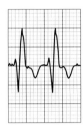

R^1 taller than R peak in lead V_1

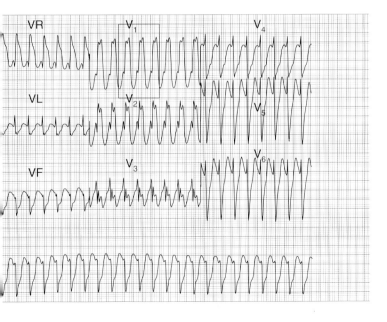

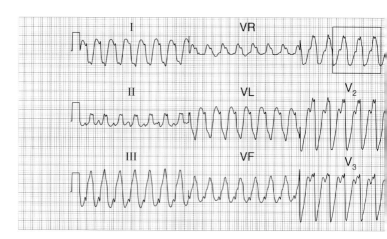

Fig. 3.58 Post-cardioversion: sinus rhythm with normal conduction

Note

- Same patient as in Figure 3.57
- Sinus rhythm
- Axis now shows left deviation
- Narrow QRS complexes
- Widespread ST segment depression, indicating ischaemia
- The narrow QRS complexes, with a change of axis, show that the original rhythm (shown in Fig. 3.57) must have been ventricular

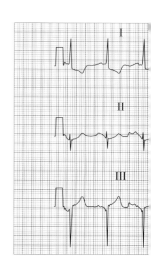

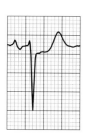

Narrow QRS complexes in lead V₁

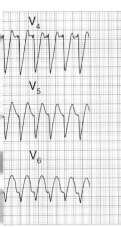

Fig. 3.57 Broad complex tachycardia, ?ventricular, ?supraventricular

Note
- Regular rhythm at 180/min
- Right axis deviation
- Very broad complexes with QRS duration 200 ms
- R and R^1 peaks are variable
- No concordance

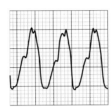

Variable R and R^1 peaks in lead V$_1$

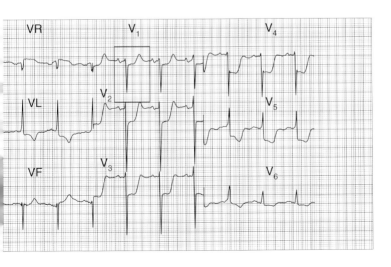

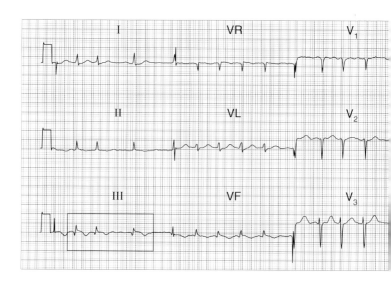

Fig. 3.60 Ventricular tachycardia and inferior infarction

Note

- Same patient as in Figure 3.59
- Broad complex tachycardia
- Intermediate axis
- RBBB pattern, but R peak greater than R^1 in lead V_1
- No concordance
- With acute myocardial infarction this will be VT

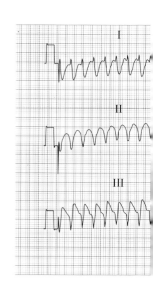

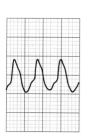

RBBB pattern in lead V_1

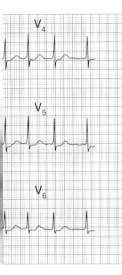

Fig. 3.59 Atrial fibrillation and inferior infarction

Note

- Irregular, narrow complex rhythm
- Irregular baseline indicates atrial fibrillation
- Small Q waves in leads III and VF with inverted T waves, suggest inferior infarction
- Slight ST segment depression in leads V_4–V_5 suggests ischaemia

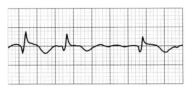

Small Q waves and inverted T waves in lead III

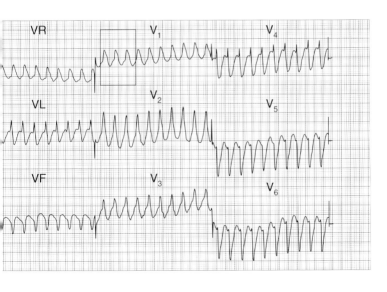

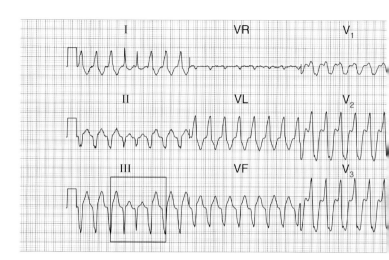

Fusion beats and capture beats

If an early beat can be found with a narrow QRS complex, it can be assumed that a wide complex tachycardia is ventricular in origin. The narrow early beat demonstrates that the bundle branches will conduct supraventricular beats normally, even at high heart rates.

A 'fusion beat' is said to occur when the ventricles are activated simultaneously by a supraventricular and a ventricular impulse, so that a QRS complex with an intermediate pattern is seen (Fig. 3.61). A 'capture beat' occurs when the ventricles are activated by an impulse of supraventricular origin during a run of VT.

Figure 3.62 shows another example of a capture beat, indicating that the broad complex tachycardia is VT.

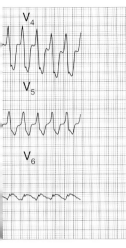

Fig. 3.61 Ventricular tachycardia

Note
- Broad complex tachycardia at 180/min
- Left axis deviation
- Probable RBBB pattern, with R peak greater than R^1
- Two narrow complexes in leads I, II and III – the first is probably a 'fusion' beat and the second a 'capture' beat

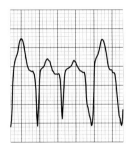

Fusion and capture beats in lead III

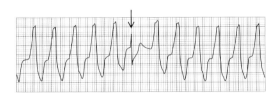

Fig. 3.62 Ventricular tachycardia

Note
- A single early beat with a narrow QRS complex (arrowed) interrupts a broad complex tachycardia
- A single 'capture' beat must have a supraventricular origin, and by inference the broad complexes must have a ventricular origin

Special forms of ventricular tachycardia in patients with symptoms

Right ventricular outflow tract tachycardia
This is usually an exercise-induced tachycardia, which originates in the right ventricular outflow tract. It can be treated by ablation. It is recognizable because the broad complex tachycardia shows the combination of right axis deviation and an LBBB (Fig. 3.63).

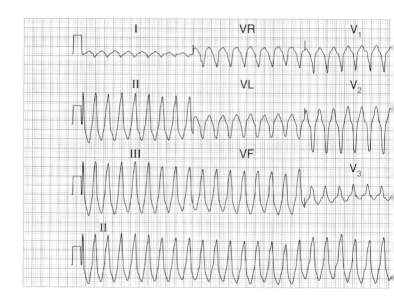

Torsade de pointes

VT is called 'monomorphic' when all the QRS complexes have the same appearance, and 'polymorphic' when they vary. A 'twisting' polymorphic VT is called 'torsade de pointes'. This is associated with a long QT interval (see p. 129) when the tachycardia is not present. Figures 3.64 and 3.65 show the ECGs from a patient with a long QT interval when in sinus rhythm, who developed torsade de pointes VT. This pattern immediately raises the possibility of drug toxicity, and in this case the cause was thioridazine.

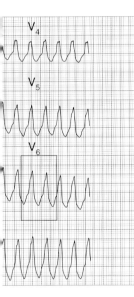

Fig. 3.63 Right ventricular outflow tract tachycardia

Note
- Broad complex tachycardia
- Right axis deviation
- LBBB pattern

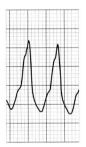

Broad QRS complexes and LBBB pattern in lead V_6

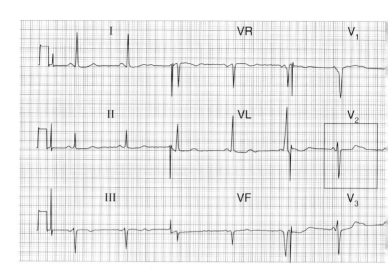

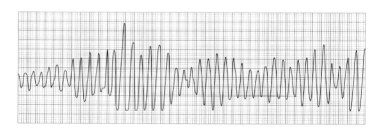

Fig. 3.65 Torsade de pointes ventricular tachycardia

Note
• Broad complex, polymorphic tachycardia with continual change of shape

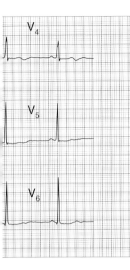

Fig. 3.64 Long QT syndrome: drug toxicity

Note
- Sinus rhythm
- Third complex in lead VL is probably a 'fusion' beat
- QT interval difficult to measure because of U waves, but probably about 540 ms

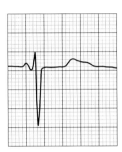

Long QT interval in lead V_2

Broad complex tachycardias associated with Wolff–Parkinson–White syndrome

Remember that the WPW syndrome causes a wide QRS complex because of the delta wave. When a re-entry tachycardia occurs with depolarization down the accessory pathway, the ECG will show a wide QRS complex which can look remarkably like VT. When the broad complex tachycardia is polymorphic (variable-shape QRS complexes) and very irregular, the rhythm is likely to be atrial fibrillation with the WPW syndrome. This is extremely dangerous, as it can degenerate to ventricular fibrillation (Figs 3.66 and 3.67).

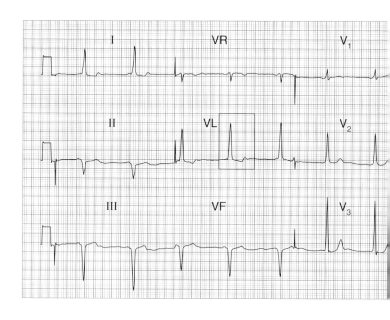

Fig. 3.67 Wolff–Parkinson–White syndrome with atrial fibrillation

Note

- Same patient as in Figure 3.66
- Irregular broad complex tachycardia
- Rate up to 300/min
- Delta waves still apparent
- Marked irregularity suggests AF

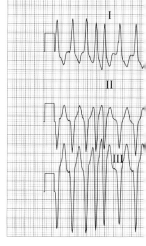

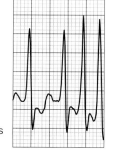

Delta waves in lead V₂

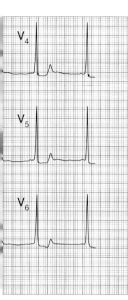

Fig. 3.66 Wolff–Parkinson–White syndrome

Note
- Sinus rhythm
- Short PR interval
- Left axis deviation
- Prominent delta wave
- Dominant R waves in lead V_1

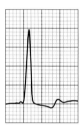

Short PR interval and delta wave in lead VL

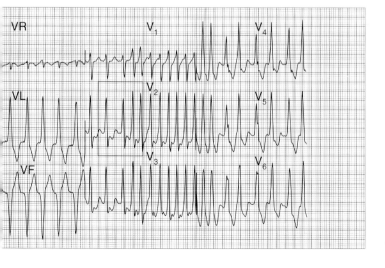

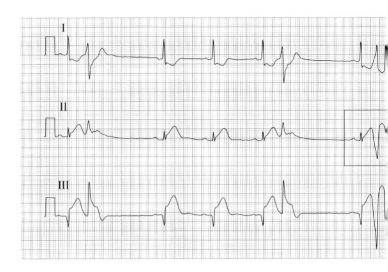

Ventricular fibrillation
The ECG in Figure 3.68 was being recorded from a patient with an acute inferior myocardial infarction when he collapsed due to VF.

Bradycardias in patients with symptoms

Escape rhythms
The pathophysiology of the escape rhythms has been discussed in Chapter 1. Escape rhythms are usually asymptomatic, but symptoms occur when the automaticity that generates the escape rhythm is inadequate to maintain a cardiac output.

Sinoatrial disease – the 'sick sinus syndrome'
Abnormal function of the SA node may be associated with failure of the conduction system. Many patients with sinoatrial disease are asymptomatic, but all the symptoms associated with bradycardias – dizziness, syncope and the symptoms of heart failure – can occur.

The abnormal rhythms seen in the sick sinus syndrome include:

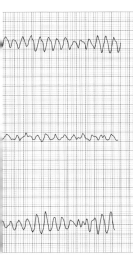

Fig. 3.68 Ventricular fibrillation

Note
- Leads I, II and III, continuous records
- Initially sinus rhythm, with occasional ventricular extrasystoles
- 'R on T' ventricular extrasystole (see p. 155) followed by VF

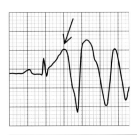

R on T phenomenon in lead II

- Unexplained or inappropriate sinus bradycardia
- Sudden changes in sinus rate
- Sinus pauses (sinoatrial arrest or exit block)
- Atrial standstill ('silent atrium')
- Atrioventricular junctional escape rhythms
- Atrial tachycardia alternating with junctional escape
- Junctional tachycardia alternating with junctional escape
- Atrial fibrillation with a slow ventricular response
- Prolonged pauses after premature atrial beats.

Disordered SA node function can be familial or congenital and can occur in ischaemic, rheumatic, hypertensive or infiltrative cardiac disease. It is, however, frequently idiopathic. Because atrial and junctional tachycardias often occur together, the patient may present with palpitations. The combination of sick sinus syndrome and tachycardias is sometimes called the 'bradycardia–tachycardia syndrome'. The ECGs in Figures 3.69 and 3.70 are from a young man who had a normal ECG with a slow sinus rate when asymptomatic, but who intermittently became extremely dizzy when he developed a profound sinus bradycardia.

199

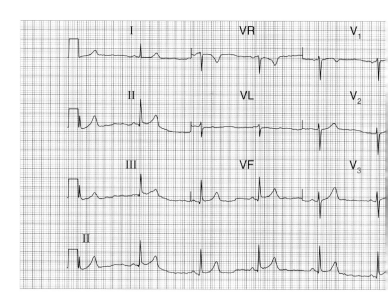

Fig. 3.70 Sick sinus syndrome: sinus bradycardia

Note
- Same patient as in Figure 3.69
- Sinus rhythm
- Rate down to 12/min at times
- No complexes recorded in leads V_1–V_3

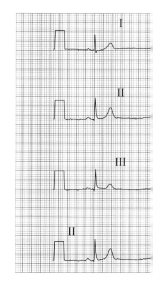

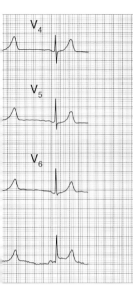

Fig. 3.69 Sinus bradycardia

Note
- Sinus rhythm
- Rate 45/min, ECG otherwise normal

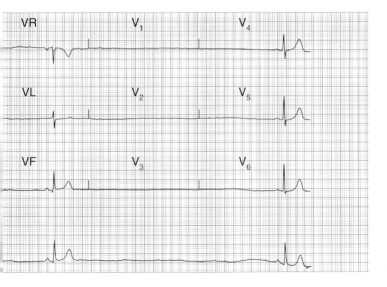

The ECG in Figure 3.71 shows an ambulatory record from a young woman who complained of short-lived attacks of dizziness. When she had these, the ECG showed sinus pauses.

The ECG in Figure 3.72 shows an example of a 'silent atrium', when the heart rhythm depends on the irregular depolarization of a focus in the AV node.

Figure 3.73 shows the rhythm of a patient with the 'bradycardia–tachycardia' syndrome. This patient was asymptomatic at times when his ECG shows a 'silent atrium' with a slow and irregular junctional (AV nodal) escape rhythm, but complained of palpitations when he had an AV nodal tachycardia.

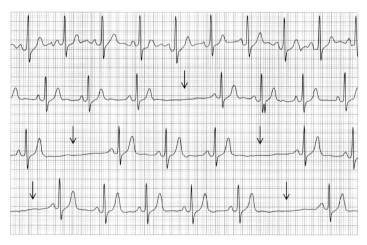

Fig. 3.71 Sinus pauses

Note
- Ambulatory record
- Sinus rhythm throughout, but marked pauses (arrowed) at time of symptoms

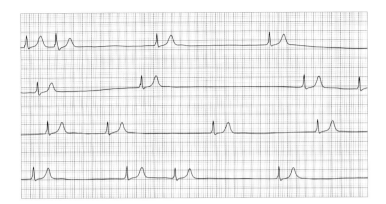

Fig. 3.72 Sick sinus syndrome: silent atrium

Note
- Ambulatory recording from lead II
- Irregular, narrow complex rhythm
- No P waves visible
- Nodal escape, with rate down to 16/min at times

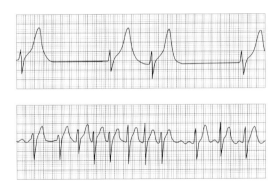

Fig. 3.73 Sick sinus syndrome: bradycardia–tachycardia syndrome

Note
- Upper trace: a silent atrium with irregular junctional escape beats
- Lower trace: junctional tachycardia is followed by a period of sinus rhythm

203

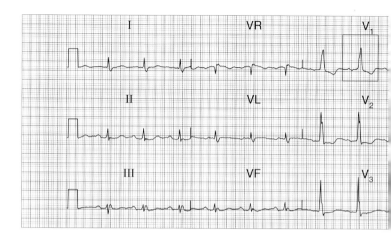

Figure 3.74 shows the ECG from a patient who, when asymptomatic, showed first degree block and RBBB. He complained of fainting attacks, and an ambulatory recording (Fig. 3.75) showed that this was due to sinus arrest with a very slow AV nodal escape rhythm, giving a ventricular rate of 15/min. This is an example of the combination of conduction system disease and sick sinus syndrome.

Atrial fibrillation and flutter
A slow ventricular rate can accompany atrial flutter or atrial fibrillation because of slow conduction through the AV node and His bundle systems (Figs. 3.76 and 3.77). This may be the result of treatment with drugs that delay AV nodal conduction, such as digoxin, beta-blockers or verapamil, but can occur because of conducting tissue disease.

Complete block associated with atrial fibrillation is recognized from the regular and wide QRS complexes which originate in the ventricular muscle (Fig. 3.78).

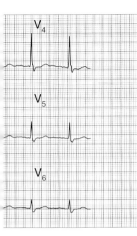

Fig. 3.74 First degree block and right bundle branch block

Note
- Sinus rhythm
- PR interval 220 ms (first degree block)
- RBBB

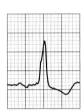

Long PR interval and RBBB pattern in lead V₁

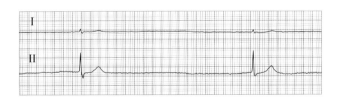

Fig. 3.75 Sinus arrest and atrioventricular nodal escape

Note
- Ambulatory record
- No P waves
- Narrow complex rhythm
- Rate 15/min, due to AV nodal (junctional) escape

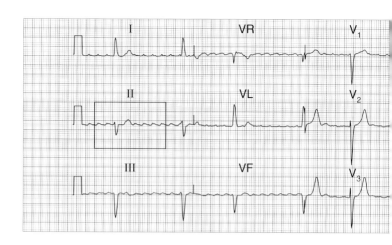

Fig. 3.77 Atrial fibrillation

Note
- Irregular rhythm, rate 43/min
- Flutter-like waves in lead V_1 but these are not constant
- Left axis deviation
- QRS complexes otherwise normal
- Prolonged QT intervals of 530 ms: ?hypokalaemia

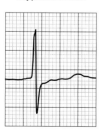

Prolonged QT interval in lead V_4

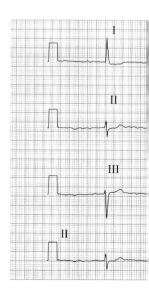

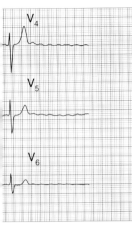

Fig. 3.76 Atrial flutter with variable block

Note
- Irregular bradycardia
- Flutter waves at 300/min obvious in all leads
- Ventricular rate varies, range 30–55/min
- QRS complex duration slightly prolonged (128 ms), indicating partial RBBB
- There is not complete block, as shown by the irregular QRS complexes

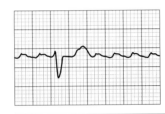

Flutter waves in lead II

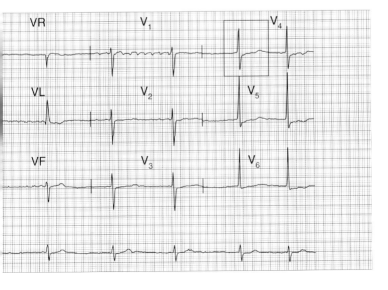

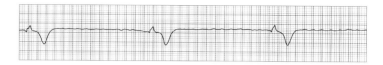

Fig. 3.78 Atrial fibrillation and complete block

Note
- Irregular baseline suggests atrial fibrillation
- Regular broad complexes, rate about 15/min
- Inverted T waves

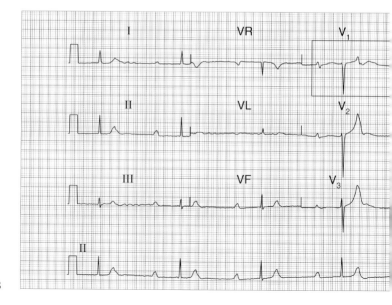

Atrioventricular block
Symptoms are not caused by first degree block, second degree
block of the Wenckebach and Mobitz type 2 varieties, left anterior
hemiblock or the bundle branch blocks.

2:1 second degree block will cause dizziness and breathlessness
if the ventricular rate is slow enough (Fig. 3.79). Young people
tolerate slower hearts than old people.

Complete (third degree) block characteristically has a slow
rate, but this may be fast enough to cause only tiredness or the
symptoms of heart failure. Figure 3.80 shows the ECG of a 60-year-
old man who, despite a heart rate of 40/min, had few complaints.

If the ventricular rate is very slow the patient may lose
consciousness in a 'Stokes–Adams' attack, which can cause a
seizure and sometimes death. The ECG in Figure 3.81 was from
a patient who was asymptomatic while his ECG showed sinus
rhythm with first degree block and RBBB but who then had a
Stokes–Adams attack with the onset of complete block (Fig. 3.82).

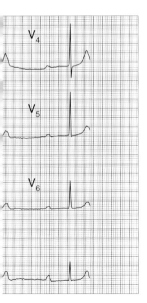

Fig. 3.79 Second degree block (2:1)

Note
- Sinus rhythm
- Second degree block, 2:1 type
- Ventricular rate 33/min
- Normal QRS complexes and T waves

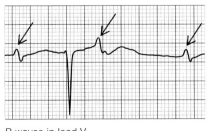

P waves in lead V_1

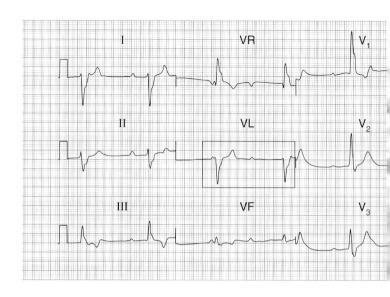

Fig. 3.81 First degree block and right bundle branch block

Note
- Sinus rhythm
- PR interval 240 ms
- Right axis deviation
- RBBB

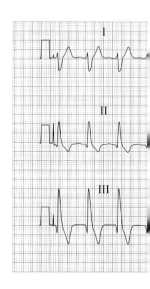

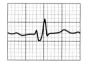

Long PR interval and RBBB pattern in lead V_1

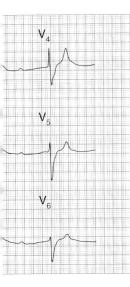

Fig. 3.80 Complete heart block

Note

- Sinus rate 70/min
- Regular ventricular rate, 40/min
- No relationship between P waves and QRS complexes
- Wide QRS complexes
- RBBB pattern

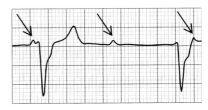

P waves in lead VL

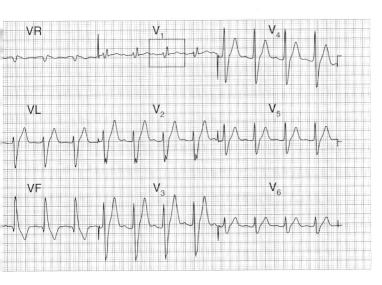

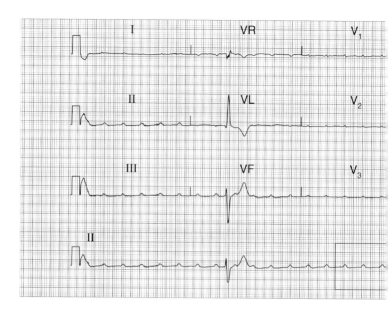

AMBULATORY ECG RECORDING

The only way to be certain that a patient's symptoms are due to an arrhythmia is to show that an arrhythmia is present at the time. If symptoms occur frequently – say two or three times a week – a 24-hour tape recording (called a 'Holter' record after its inventor) may show the abnormality. When symptoms are infrequent, patient-activated 'event recorders' are more useful.

Figures 3.83, 3.84, and 3.85 show examples of ambulatory records obtained from patients who complained of syncopal attacks, but whose hearts were in sinus rhythm at the time they were seen.

When an ambulatory record shows arrhythmias which are not accompanied by symptoms, it is difficult to be certain of their significance. Table 3.6 shows the arrhythmias that were recorded during two 24-hour periods from a group of 86 volunteers who were apparently completely free of heart disease. This study shows that supposedly dangerous arrhythmias, such as VT, can occur and pass unnoticed in apparently healthy people.

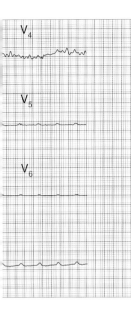

Fig. 3.82 Complete block and Stokes–Adams attack

Note

- Same patient as in Figure 3.81
- Sinus rate 140/min
- Ventricular rate 15/min
- No relationship between P waves and QRS complexes
- No QRS complexes recorded in leads I, II, III, V$_1$–V$_3$

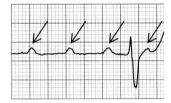

P waves

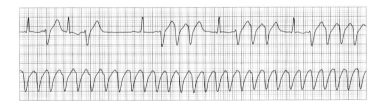

Fig. 3.83 Ventricular tachycardia

Note

- Ambulatory recording
- Initially sinus rhythm with ventricular extrasystoles
- Then salvos (three beats) of extrasystoles, leading to a broad complex tachycardia
- The change in QRS configuration suggests that the tachycardia is ventricular but a 12-lead ECG would be necessary to be certain

213

Ventricular extrasystoles are so common that they can clearly be ignored, although epidemiological evidence suggests that in large groups of patients they can be crude 'markers' of heart disease.

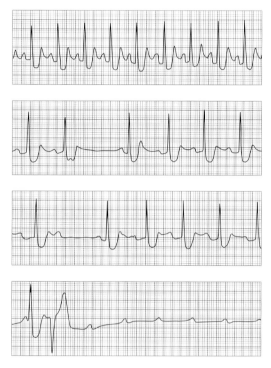

Fig. 3.84 Ventricular standstill

Note

- Ambulatory recording
- Top strip shows sinus rhythm with normal AV conduction
- Second strip shows SA block, which was also asymptomatic
- Third strip shows second degree block, which was asymptomatic
- Bottom strip shows a ventricular extrasystole followed by ventricular standstill. The patient lost consciousness due to this Stokes–Adams attack

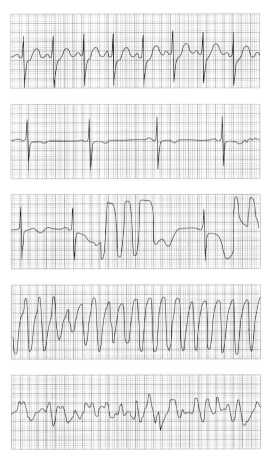

Fig. 3.85 Sudden death due to ventricular fibrillation

Note
- Ambulatory recording
- First strip shows sinus rhythm
- Sinus bradycardia then develops, with inversion of the T wave suggesting ischaemia
- Short runs of VT lead to polymorphic ventricular tachycardia
- Ventricular fibrillation then develops

Table 3.6 Arrhythmias observed during 48 hours of ambulatory recording in 86 healthy subjects aged 16-65 (from Clarke et al 1976 Lancet 2:508–510)

Type of arrhythmia	No. of individuals with arrhythmia		
Ventricular extrasystoles	63	(including: multifocal	13
		bigeminy	13
		R on T	3)
Ventricular tachycardia	2		
Supraventricular tachycardia	4		
Junctional escape	8		
Second degree block	2		

THE ECG IN PATIENTS WITH PACEMAKERS

The presence of a pacemaker in a recording can be identified by the presence of a sharp pacing 'spike', which may precede the

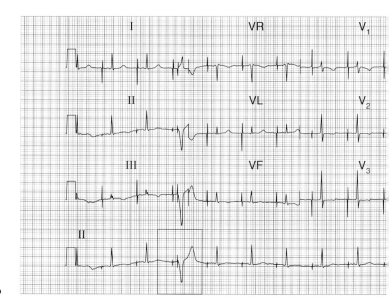

P wave if the atrium is paced, or the QRS complex if the ventricle is paced.

Atrial pacing is used in the sick sinus syndrome and in patients without any conduction disturbance. The QRS complex remains normal. Ventricular pacing is necessary for patients with complete heart block. The pacing catheter is in the right ventricle, effectively producing ventricular beats, so the QRS complex is wide and abnormal.

Pacemakers sense intrinsic cardiac activity, and when this occurs pacing is inhibited. An ECG may therefore show a mixture of paced and normal beats.

Ensuring that atrial depolarization is appropriately followed by ventricular depolarization makes the heart more efficient than simple ventricular pacing. This can be achieved either by sequential pacing of the right atrium and ventricle, or by sensing atrial depolarization and stimulating the ventricle after an appropriate delay. Figures 3.86, 3.87, 3.88, 3.89 and 3.90 show examples of ECGs of patients with pacemakers.

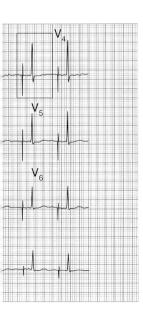

Fig. 3.86 Atrial pacing

Note
- Pacing spike precedes P waves
- Narrow QRS complexes
- The third beat shows atrial and ventricular pacing

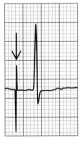

Pacing spike in lead V_4

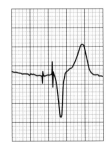

Atrial then ventricular pacing spikes

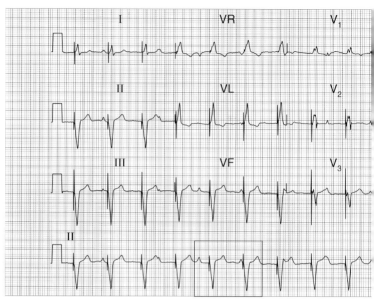

Fig. 3.88 Ventricular pacing

Note

- Ventricular pacing
- Underlying rhythm can be seen to be atrial fibrillation
- Final two beats with narrow complexes are not paced – the intrinsic heart rate exceeds that of the pacemaker and the pacemaker is inhibited

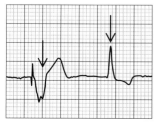

First beat paced, second beat unpaced

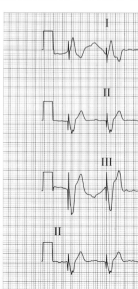

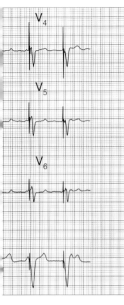

Fig. 3.87 Ventricular pacing

Note
- Ventricular pacing
- P waves can be seen, unrelated to ventricular beats
- Therefore the underlying rhythm is complete heart block

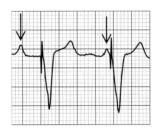

Complete block (P waves arrowed)

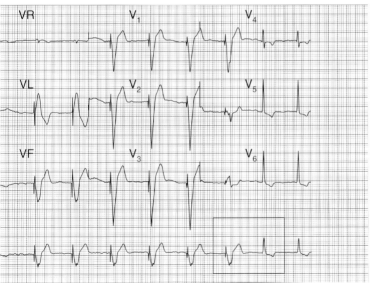

219

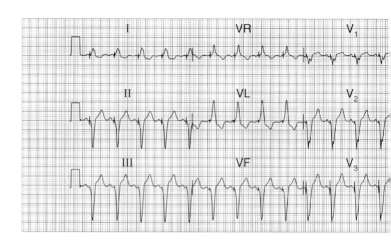

Fig. 3.90 Dual chamber pacing

Note

• A pacing spike can be seen before each
  P wave and before each QRS complex

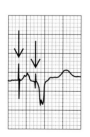

Atrial pacing followed
by ventricular pacing
in lead II

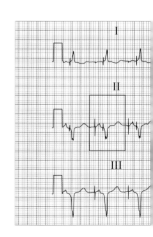

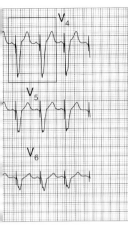

Fig. 3.89 Atrial sensing, ventricular pacing

Note
- A pacing spike can be seen in front of each wide QRS complex
- There is a P wave before each pacing spike
- The pacemaker must have sensed the P wave and coupled the QRS complex to it

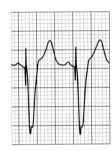

Pacing spike following P wave in lead V₄

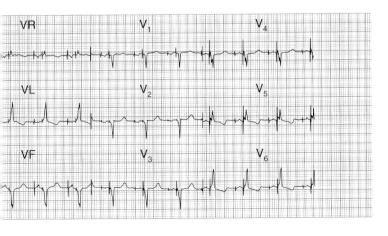

WHAT TO DO

What to do when an arrhythmia is suspected

Precipitation of arrhythmias

Arrhythmias are sometimes precipitated by exercise (Fig. 3.91) and if the patient's history suggests that this is so, then treadmill testing may be helpful. Attempts to provoke an arrhythmia by exercise should, however, only be made when full resuscitation facilities are available.

   If the patient complains of syncopal attacks, particularly on movement of the head, it is worth pressing the carotid sinus in the neck to see if the patient has carotid sinus hypersensitivity. Complete SA node inhibition may be induced, sometimes with unpleasant effects (Fig. 3.92).

Rest

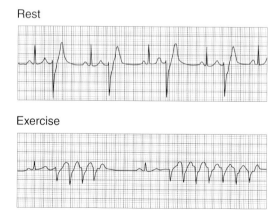

Exercise

Fig. 3.91 Exercise-induced ventricular tachycardia

Note
- At rest (upper trace) the ECG shows frequent ventricular extrasystoles
- During exercise (lower trace), VT occurs

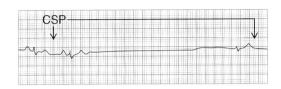

Fig. 3.92 Carotid sinus hypersensitivity

Note
- Carotid sinus pressure (CSP) causes cessation of all cardiac activity, due to excessive vagal influence

What to do when an arrhythmia is recorded
First ask:

1. Does the arrhythmia need treating as an emergency?
   - If there are unpleasant symptoms, or evidence of haemodynamic disturbance – yes
   - If the patient is asymptomatic – probably not, unless haemodynamic problems seem likely.
2. Does the arrhythmia have an obvious cause? Possible causes are:
   - Myocardial infarction, sometimes following thrombolysis (not usually important)
   - Drugs (especially antiarrhythmic drugs)
   - Alcohol
   - Thyrotoxicosis
   - Rheumatic heart disease
   - Cardiomyopathy.

What follows is a simple and safe therapeutic policy, based on a few drugs, for arrhythmias that need treating.

Principles of arrhythmia management
- Any arrhythmia causing significant symptoms or a haemodynamic disturbance must be treated immediately.
- All antiarrhythmic drugs should be considered cardiac depressants, and they are potentially pro-arrhythmic. The use of multiple agents should be avoided.

- Electrical treatment (cardioversion for tachycardias, pacing for bradycardias) should be used in preference to drug therapy when there is marked haemodynamic impairment.

Management of cardiac arrest

The treatment of an individual patient will depend on the particular arrhythmia involved. Remember, confirm cardiac arrest by checking:

- Airway
- Breathing
- Circulation.

The immediate actions are:

- Begin cardiopulmonary resuscitation (CPR). Ventilation and chest compression should be given in a ratio of 2 breaths to every 15 compressions.
- Defibrillate in cases of VF and pulseless ventricular tachycardia as soon as possible.
- Intubate as soon as possible.
- Gain or verify IV access.

Ventricular fibrillation or pulseless ventricular tachycardia (pVT)
Actions:

1. Precordial thump (especially useful in VT)
2. Defibrillate at 200 J
3. If unsuccessful, repeat defibrillation at 200 J
4. If unsuccessful, defibrillation at 360 J
5. If unsuccessful, give adrenaline (epinephrine) 1 mg i.v.
6. 1 min of CPR
7. If VF/pVT persists, give amiodarone 300 mg i.v.
8. Defibrillate at 360 J
9. Defibrillate at 360 J
10. Defibrillate at 360 J
11. If still unsuccessful, repeat 1 min of CPR and defibrillate again
12. Give adrenaline (epinephrine) 1 mg i.v. every 3 min.

The ECG in Figure 3.93 shows a successful defibrillation.

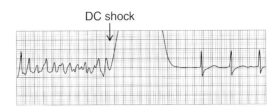

Fig. 3.93 DC conversion of ventricular fibrillation

Note
- VF is abolished by DC shock
- A supraventricular rhythm (probably sinus in origin) immediately takes control of the heart

Asystole and pulseless electrical activity (PEA)
The term PEA now replaces 'electromechanical dissociation' (EMD) because some pulseless patients have some weak myocardial contractions, although insufficient to generate a cardiac output. Actions:

1. Precordial thump
2. If it is unclear whether the rhythm is 'fine VF' or asystole, treat as VF until three defibrillations have not changed the apparent rhythm.
3. Adrenaline (epinephrine) 1 mg i.v.
4. Atropine 3 mg i.v.
5. 3 min of CPR
6. If unsuccessful, continue adrenaline (epinephrine) 1 mg and CPR in 3 min cycles
7. Consider the possibility of a treatable cause:
   - Hypoxia
   - Hypovolaemia
   - Hyperkalaemia, hypocalcaemia, acidaemia
   - Hypothermia
   - Tension pneumothorax
   - Cardiac tamponade
   - Toxic substances, or therapeutic substances in overdose
   - Thromboembolic or mechanical obstruction (e.g. pulmonary embolus).

225

Following resuscitation, check:

- Arterial blood gases – if the pH is < 7.1 or if arrest is associated with tricyclic overdose, give bicarbonate 50 mmol.
- Electrolytes
- ECG
- Chest X-ray – principally to exclude a pneumothorax caused by the resuscitation.

It is not necessary to give routine antiarrhythmic therapy after a successful resuscitation.

Management of other arrhythmias

Extrasystoles
Supraventricular: no treatment. If the patient has symptoms, explanation and reassurance.

Ventricular: usually no treatment, though treatment may be considered:

- when ventricular extrasystoles are so frequent that cardiac output is impaired
- when there is a frequent R on T phenomenon
- when the patient complains of an irregular heartbeat but reassurance and an explanation prove ineffective.

Three ventricular extrasystoles together (a 'salvo') should be treated as a ventricular tachycardia.

Carotid sinus pressure in the management of tachycardias
The first step in the management of any tachycardia is to try CSP.
In sinus rhythm, CSP will cause transient slowing of the heart rate. This may be useful in identifying the true origin of the rhythm when there is doubt (Fig. 3.94).
In atrial flutter, AV conduction is blocked so the ventricular rate falls. The atrial activity becomes obvious, which helps to identify the rhythm (Fig. 3.95). CSP seldom converts atrial flutter to sinus rhythm.

Without CSP

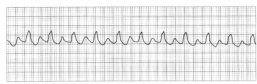

With CSP

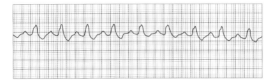

Fig. 3.94 CSP and sinus rhythm

Note
- Upper trace shows a broad complex tachycardia
- It is not obvious whether the deflection before the QRS complex represents a T wave or a T wave followed by a P wave
- Lower trace shows that with CSP the rate falls, and P waves become obvious

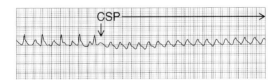

Fig. 3.95 CSP in atrial flutter

Note

- CSP increases the block at the AV node
- Ventricular activity is completely suppressed
- 'Flutter' waves are obvious

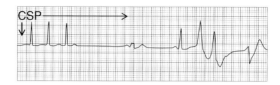

Fig. 3.96 CSP in junctional tachycardia

Note
• CSP reverts junctional tachycardia to sinus rhythm, but in this case multifocal ventricular extrasystoles occurred

---

In atrial tachycardia and junctional tachycardia, CSP may restore sinus rhythm (Fig. 3.96).

In atrial fibrillation and VT, CSP has no effect.

Sinus tachycardia
Remember that sinus tachycardia always has a cause (see Table 3.4, p. 115), and it is the cause that should be treated.

Atrioventricular re-entry (junctional) tachycardia
Try in order:

1. Carotid sinus massage
2. Adenosine 3 mg i.v. bolus, followed if necessary after 2 min by a further 6 mg adenosine and, if necessary after a further 2 min, by a further 12 mg adenosine. Unwanted but transient effects include asthma, flushing, chest tightness and dizziness.
3. Verapamil 5–10 mg i.v. or atenolol 2.5 mg i.v., repeated at 5 min intervals to a total of 10 mg. NB: These drugs should not be administered together and verapamil should not be given to patients receiving a beta-blocker.
4. DC shock

Atrial tachycardia
Remember that this may be due to digoxin toxicity. Treat as for junctional tachycardia.

Atrial fibrillation and flutter
A choice has to be made between rate control and conversion of atrial fibrillation to sinus rhythm. It should be remembered that long-term success following conversion is very unlikely in patients who:

- have had atrial fibrillation for more than a year
- have cardiac enlargement
- have evidence of left ventricular impairment
- have any form of structural abnormality in the heart.

If a patient has a ventricular rate > 150/min and chest pain or other evidence of poor perfusion, immediate cardioversion should be attempted. In an emergency, immediate heparin provides adequate prophylaxis against embolism. Cardioversion can be attempted with amiodarone i.v. or flecainide i.v., but electrical cardioversion (100 J – 200 J – 360 J) is more reliable.

Patients who are not haemodynamically impaired, and who have been in atrial fibrillation for more than 24 h, should be treated with warfarin before cardioversion is attempted. Effective anticoagulation (INR > 2.0) is needed for at least 1 month before the procedure.

For rate control, use one of:

- digoxin 250 µg i.v. by slow injection, repeated at 30 min intervals to a total of 1 mg
- i.v. verapamil
- i.v. beta-blocker
- i.v. amiodarone

and remember the need for anticoagulants.

Prevention of paroxysmal atrial fibrillation. Atrial fibrillation is called 'paroxysmal' if there are attacks that revert spontaneously; 'persistent' if the rhythm is continuous but cardioversion has not been attempted; and 'permanent' if cardioversion has failed.

Digoxin will probably not prevent attacks of atrial fibrillation, but the prophylactic use of some drugs may prevent attacks for months, or possibly years:

- sotalol
- flecainide (avoid in patients with coronary disease)
- amiodarone.

These drugs can be used after DC cardioversion, but at best only about 40% of patients will still be in sinus rhythm after a year.

In very resistant cases, electrical ablation of the AV node can be used to cause complete heart block, and a permanent pacemaker inserted.

Ventricular tachycardia

Ventricular tachycardia is a broad complex tachycardia occurring with a heart rate exceeding 120/min. It can be treated with one of:

- lidocaine (lignocaine) 100 mg i.v., repeated twice at 5 min intervals, followed by a lidocaine infusion at 2–3 mg/min
- amiodarone 300 mg i.v. over 30 min then 900 mg over 24 h, followed by 200 mg t.d.s. by mouth for 1 week, 200 mg b.d. for 1 week and 200 mg daily thereafter
- atenolol 2.5 mg i.v., repeated at 5 min intervals to 10 mg
- flecainide 50–100 mg i.v., or 100 mg b.d. by mouth – but avoid in patients with coronary disease
- magnesium 8 mmol i.v. over 15 min, followed by 64 mmol over 24 h.

NB: When amiodarone is given i.v. a deep vein must be used. Overdose prolongs the QT interval and can cause tachycardia. Long-term treatment may cause skin pigmentation, photosensitive rashes, abnormalities of thyroid or liver function, drug deposits in the cornea, or, occasionally, pulmonary fibrosis.

Second-line drugs for ventricular tachycardia include disopyramide and mexiletine. Recurrent episodes, which cannot be controlled by drugs, are treated with an implanted defibrillator.

Patients with congenital long QT syndromes and paroxysmal ventricular tachycardia are treated in the first instance with beta-blockers, or with an implanted defibrillator.

Wolff–Parkinson–White syndrome
Adenosine, digoxin, verapamil and lidocaine (lignocaine) may increase conduction through the accessory pathway and block it in the AV node. This can be extremely dangerous if atrial fibrillation occurs, because it may lead to VF. These drugs should therefore not be used for the treatment of pre-excitation tachycardias.

Drugs that slow conduction in the accessory pathway are:

- atenolol
- flecainide
- amiodarone.

These drugs can be used for prophylaxis against paroxysmal arrhythmias, but the definitive treatment is electrical ablation of the accessory pathway.

Bradycardias
Bradycardias must be treated if they are associated with hypotension, poor peripheral perfusion, or escape arrhythmias. Any bradycardia can be treated with:

- atropine 600 µg i.v., repeated at 5 min intervals to a total of 1.8 mg. NB: Overdose causes tachycardia, hallucinations and urinary retention.
- isoprenaline 1–4 µg/min. NB: Overdose causes ventricular arrhythmias which are difficult to treat. An isoprenaline infusion should only be used while preparations are being made for pacing.

Temporary pacing in patients with acute myocardial infarction. Pacing should be performed under the following circumstances:

- Complete block with ventricular rate < 50/min
- Complete block with anterior infarction
- Any persistent bradycardia needing an isoprenaline infusion
- Bifascicular block plus first degree block.

Pacing should be considered in:

- Any complete block
- Second degree block with heart rate < 50/min
- Bundle branch block plus first degree block
- Evidence of increasing block
- Bradycardia with escape rhythms
- Drug-induced tachyarrhythmias.

4

The ECG in patients with chest pain

HISTORY AND EXAMINATION

There are many causes of chest pain. All the non-cardiac conditions can mimic a myocardial infarction, and so the ECG can be extremely useful when making a diagnosis. However, the ECG is less important than the history and physical examination, because the ECG can be normal in the first few hours of a myocardial infarction.

Acute chest pain can be caused by:

- Myocardial infarction
- Pulmonary embolism
- Pneumothorax
- Other causes of pleuritic pain
- Pericarditis
- Aortic dissection

233

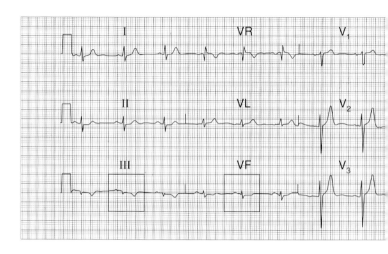

- Ruptured oesophagus
- Oesophagitis
- Collapsed vertebra
- Herpes zoster.

Chronic or *recurrent* chest pain may be:

- Angina
- Nerve root pain
- Muscular pain
- Oesophageal reflux
- Nonspecific pain.

The ECG in Figure 4.1 was recorded in an A & E department from a 44-year-old man with rather vague chest pain. He was thought to have a viral illness and his ECG was considered to be within normal limits. He was allowed home, and died later that day. The postmortem examination showed a myocardial infarction which was probably a few hours old, and corresponded with his A & E attendance.

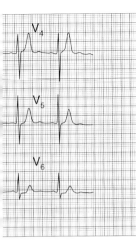

Fig. 4.1 Non-specific ST segment/T wave changes

Note
- Sinus rhythm
- Normal axis
- Normal QRS complexes
- ST segments probably normal, though possibly depressed in leads III and VF
- T wave inverted in lead III (possibly a normal variant) and flattened in VF

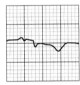

Inverted T wave
in lead III

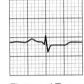

Flattened T wave
in lead VF

Acute chest pain

The typical pain of *myocardial infarction* is easy to recognize, the features being:

- central
- radiates to neck, jaw, teeth, arm(s) or back
- severe
- associated with nausea, vomiting and sweating.

Unfortunately not all patients have typical pain, and pain can even be absent.

Pulmonary embolism:

- causes pain similar to myocardial infarction if the embolus is central
- causes pleuritic pain if the embolus is peripheral
- is associated with breathlessness or haemoptysis
- can cause haemodynamic collapse.

Other lung disease, such as *infection* or *pneumothorax*, can be recognized from the pleuritic nature of the pain. This will be:

- worse on breathing
- often associated with a cough.

Pericardial pain can mimic both cardiac ischaemia and pleuritic pain, but can be recognized because it is relieved by sitting up and leaning forward.

Aortic dissection typically causes a 'tearing' pain (as opposed to the 'crushing' sensation of a myocardial infarction), and usually radiates to the back.

Oesophageal rupture follows vomiting.

Spinal pain is affected by posture, and associated root pain follows the nerve root distribution.

Shingles (herpes zoster) catches everyone out until the rash appears, although tenderness of the skin may provide a clue.

The physical examination of a patient with chest pain may reveal nothing other than the signs associated with the pain itself (anxiety, sinus tachycardia, restlessness, a cold and sweaty skin), but some specific signs are worth looking for:

- Left ventricular failure suggests myocardial infarction.
- A raised jugular venous pressure suggests myocardial infarction or pulmonary embolus.
- A pleural friction rub suggests pulmonary embolism or infection.
- A pericardial friction rub suggests pericarditis (?viral, ?secondary to myocardial infarction) or aortic dissection.
- Aortic regurgitation suggests aortic dissection.
- Unequal pulses or blood pressure in the arms suggests aortic dissection.
- Bony tenderness suggests musculoskeletal pain.

Chronic chest pain

The main differential diagnosis is between angina and the chest pain that is common in middle-aged men, but for which no clear diagnosis is usually made. This pain is sometimes called 'atypical chest pain', but this is a dangerous diagnostic label because it implies that there is a diagnosis (by implication, cardiac ischaemia) but that the symptoms are 'atypical'. Some of these pains are musculoskeletal, Tietze's syndrome of pain from the costochondral junctions being the most obvious, but in most cases the best diagnostic label is 'chest pain of unknown cause'. This indicates a possible need for later re-evaluation.

The important features in the history that point to a diagnosis of angina are that the pain:

- is predictable
- usually occurs after a constant amount of exercise
- is worse in cold or windy weather
- is induced by emotional stress
- is induced by sexual intercourse
- is relieved by rest, and rapidly relieved by a short-acting nitrate.

The physical signs to look for are:

- Evidence of risk factors (high blood pressure, cholesterol deposits, signs of smoking)
- Any signs of cardiac disease (aortic stenosis, an enlarged heart, signs of heart failure)
- Anaemia
- Signs of peripheral vascular disease (which would suggest that coronary disease is also present).

THE ECG IN THE PRESENCE OF CHEST PAIN

Remember that the ECG can be normal in the early stages of a myocardial infarction. Having said that:

- An abnormal ECG is necessary to make a diagnosis of myocardial infarction before treatment is started.
- An ECG will demonstrate ischaemia in patients with angina *provided that* the patient has pain at the time the ECG is recorded.
- With pulmonary embolus there may be classical ECG changes, but these are often not present.
- With pericarditis, ECG changes, if present at all, are very nonspecific.

THE ECG IN PATIENTS WITH MYOCARDIAL INFARCTION

The diagnosis of a myocardial infarction depends on the history and examination, on the measurement of biochemical markers of cardiac muscle damage (especially the troponins) and on the ECG. A rise in troponin I or troponin T levels in patients with a history suggestive of a myocardial infarction is now taken to mean that infarction has occurred, but treatment still depends on the ECG. The term 'acute coronary syndrome' is now used to include:

- Myocardial infarction with ST segment elevation on the ECG
- Myocardial infarction (as shown by a troponin rise) with only T wave inversion or ST segment depression
- Chest pain with ischaemic ST segment depression but no troponin rise (what used to be called 'unstable angina')
- Sudden death due to coronary disease.

Stable angina and 'chest pain of unknown cause' remain entirely proper diagnostic labels for those patients who are admitted to hospital with chest pain, but for whom the term 'acute coronary syndrome' is inappropriate.

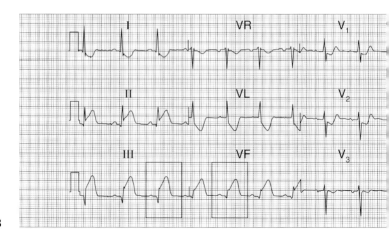

The development of ECG changes in myocardial infarction

The sequence of features characteristic of 'full thickness', or 'ST segment elevation', myocardial infarction is:

- Normal ECG
- ST segment elevation
- Development of Q waves
- ST segment returns to the baseline
- T waves become inverted.

The ECG leads that show the changes typical of a myocardial infarction depend on the part of the heart affected.

Inferior infarction
Figures 4.2, 4.3 and 4.4 show traces taken from a patient with a typical history of myocardial infarction: on admission to hospital, 3 h later, and 2 days later. The main changes are in the inferior leads II, III, and VF. Here the ST segments are initially raised, but then Q waves appear and the T waves become inverted.

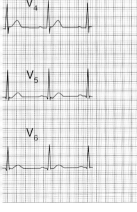

Fig. 4.2 Acute inferior infarction

Note
- Sinus rhythm
- Normal axis
- Small Q waves in leads II, III, VF
- Raised ST segments in leads II, III, VF
- Depressed ST segments in leads I, VL, V_2, V_3
- Inverted T waves in leads I, VL, V_3

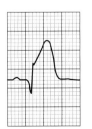 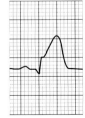

Raised ST segments in leads III and VF

239

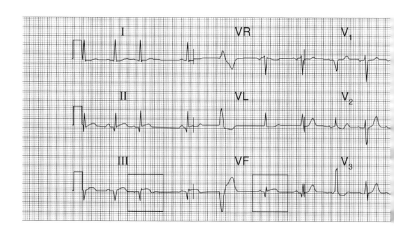

Fig. 4.4 Evolving inferior infarction

Note
- Same patient as in Figures 4.2 and 4.3
- Sinus rhythm
- Normal axis
- Q waves in leads II, III, VF
- ST segments nearly back to normal
- T wave inversion in leads II, III, VF
- Lateral ischaemia has cleared (as shown by ST segments in lateral leads)

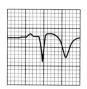 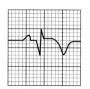

Q waves, normal ST segments, and inverted T waves in leads III and VF

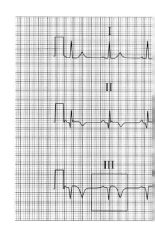

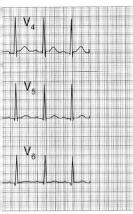

Fig. 4.3 Evolving inferior infarction

Note

- Same patient as in Figures 4.2 and 4.4
- Sinus rhythm with ventricular extrasystoles
- Normal axis
- Deeper Q waves in leads II, III, VF
- ST segments returning to normal, but still elevated in inferior leads
- Less ST segment depression in leads I, VL, V$_3$

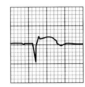 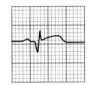

Deeper Q waves in leads III and VF

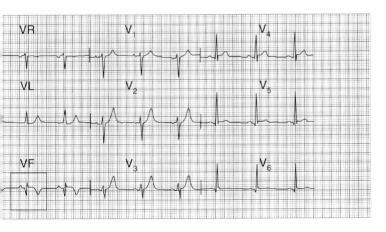

Anterior and lateral infarction

The changes of anterior infarction are seen in leads V_2–V_5. Lead V_1, which lies over the right ventricle, is seldom affected (Fig. 4.5).

The lateral wall of the left ventricle is often damaged at the same time as the anterior wall, and then leads I, VL and V_6 show infarction changes. Figures 4.6 and 4.7 show the records of a patient with an acute anterolateral infarction, initially with raised ST segments and then with T wave inversion in the lateral leads. In the ECG in Figure 4.7 left axis deviation has appeared, indicating damage to the left anterior fascicle.

Figure 4.8 shows a record taken 3 days after a lateral infarction, with Q waves and inverted T waves in leads I, VL, and V_6.

The ECG in Figure 4.9 was recorded several weeks after an anterolateral myocardial infarction. Although the changes in leads I and VL appear 'old', having an isoelectric ST segment, there is still ST segment elevation in leads V_3–V_5. If the patient had just been admitted with chest pain these changes would be taken to

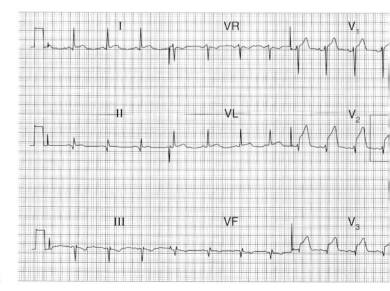

indicate an acute infarction, but this patient had had pain more than a month previously. Persistent ST segment elevation is quite common after an anterior infarction: it sometimes indicates the development of a left ventricular aneurysm, but it is not reliable evidence of this.

An old anterior infarction often causes only what is called 'poor R wave progression'. Figure 4.10 shows the record from a patient who had had an anterior infarction some years previously. A normal ECG would show progressive increase in the size of the R wave from lead V_1 to V_5 or V_6. In this case the R wave remains very small in leads V_3 and V_4, but becomes a normal size in V_5. This loss of 'progression' indicates the old infarction.

The time taken for the various ECG changes of infarction to occur is extremely variable, and the ECG is an unreliable way of deciding when an infarction occurred. Serial records showing progressive changes are the only way of timing the infarction from the ECG.

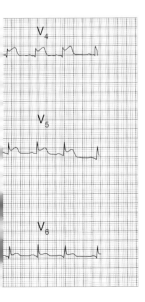

Fig. 4.5 Anterior infarction

Note
- Sinus rhythm
- Normal axis
- Raised ST segments in leads V_2–V_5

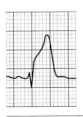

Raised ST segment in lead V_2

243

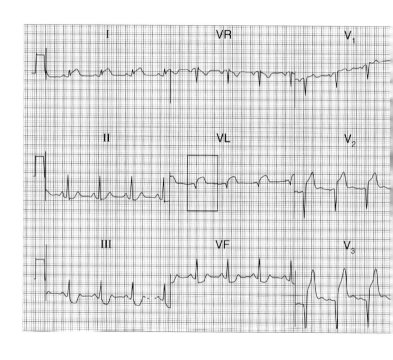

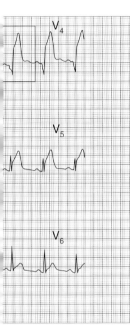

Fig. 4.6 Acute anterolateral infarction

Note
- Sinus rhythm
- Normal axis
- Q waves in leads VL, V_2–V_4
- Raised ST segments in leads I, VL, V_2–V_5

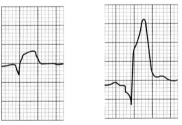

Raised ST segments in leads VL and V_4

245

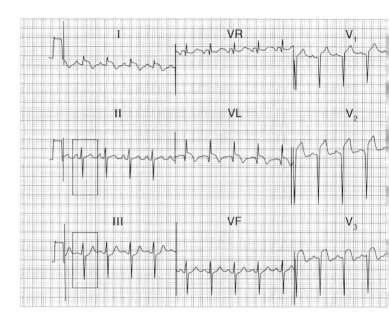

Fig. 4.8 Lateral infarction (after 3 days)

Note
- Sinus rhythm
- Normal axis
- Q waves in leads I, VL, ?V_6 (could be septal)
- ST segments isoelectric
- Inverted T waves in leads I, VL, V_6

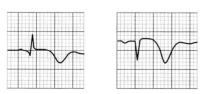

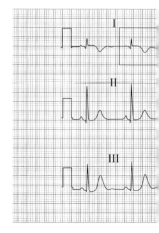

Inverted T waves in leads I and VL

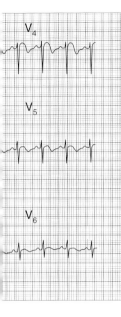

Fig. 4.7 Acute anterolateral infarction with left axis deviation

Note
- Sinus rhythm
- Left axis deviation
- ST segments now returning to normal
- T wave inversion in leads I, VL, V₄, V₅

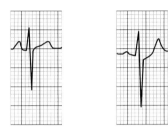

S waves in leads II and III: left axis deviation

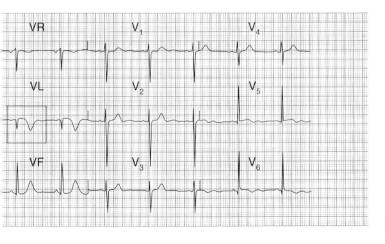

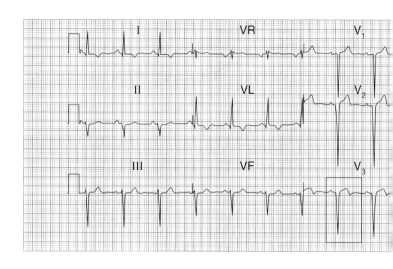

Fig. 4.10 Old anterior infarction

Note
- Sinus rhythm
- Normal axis
- Small R waves in leads V_3–V_4, large R waves in V_5: this is 'poor R wave progression'

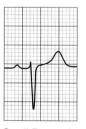

Small R wave In lead V_4

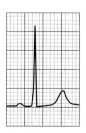

Tall R wave in lead V_5

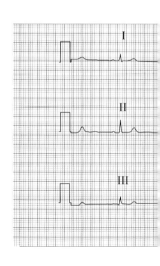

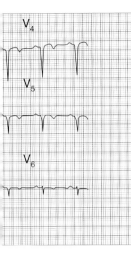

Fig. 4.9 Anterolateral infarction, ?age

Note
- Sinus rhythm
- Left axis deviation
- Q waves in leads I, II, V_2–V_5
- Raised ST segments in leads V_3–V_5
- Inverted T waves in leads I, VL, V_4–V_6

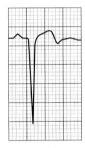

Raised ST segment in lead V_3

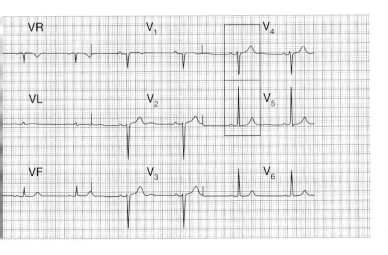

Posterior infarction

It is possible to 'look at' the back of the heart by placing the V lead on the back of the left side of the chest, but this is not done routinely because it is inconvenient and the complexes recorded are often small.

An infarction of the posterior wall of the left ventricle can, however, be detected in the ordinary 12-lead ECG because it causes a dominant R wave in lead V_1. The shape of the QRS complex recorded from lead V_1 depends on the balance of electrical forces reaching the ECG electrode. Normally the right ventricle is being depolarized towards lead V_1, so causing an upward movement (an R wave) on the record; at the same time the posterior wall of the left ventricle is being depolarized, with the wave of excitation moving away from the electrode and so

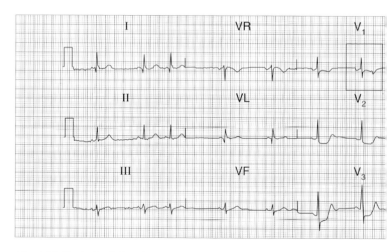

Fig. 4.11 Posterior infarction

Note
- Sinus rhythm with atrial extrasystoles
- Normal axis
- Dominant R waves in lead V_1 suggest posterior infarction
- ST segment depression in leads V_2–V_4
- Q waves and ST segment elevation in leads V_{10}–V_{12} (posterior leads)

causing a downward movement (an S wave) on the record. The left ventricle is more muscular than the right and therefore exerts a greater influence on the ECG, so in lead V_1 the QRS complex is normally predominantly downward, i.e. there is a small R wave and a deep S wave. In a posterior infarction, the rearward-moving electrical forces are lost so lead V_1 'sees' the unopposed forward-moving depolarization of the right ventricle and records a predominantly upright QRS complex.

Figure 4.11 shows the first record from a patient with acute chest pain. There is a dominant R wave in lead V_1 and ischaemic ST segment depression (see p. 267) in leads V_2–V_4. When the chest electrodes were moved to the left axilla and back, to the V_7–V_{12} positions, raised ST segments with Q waves typical of an acute infarction were seen.

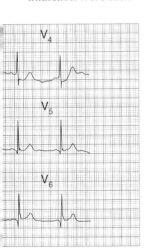

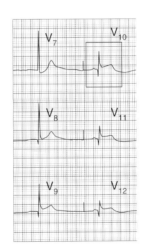

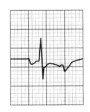

Dominant R wave in lead V_1

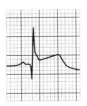

Q wave and raised ST segment in lead V_{10}

251

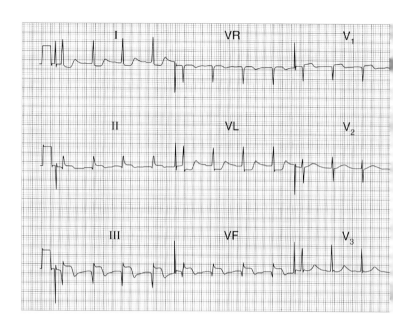

Right ventricular infarction
Inferior infarction is sometimes associated with infarction of the
right ventricle. Clinically, this is suspected in a patient with an
inferior infarction when the lungs are clear but the jugular venous
pressure is elevated. The ECG will show a raised ST segment in
leads recorded from the right side of the heart. The positions of
the leads correspond to those on the left side as follows: V_1R is in
the normal V_2 position; V_2R is in the normal V_1 position; V_3R etc.
are on the right side, in positions corresponding to V_3 etc. on the
left side. Figure 4.12 is from a patient with an acute right
ventricular infarct.

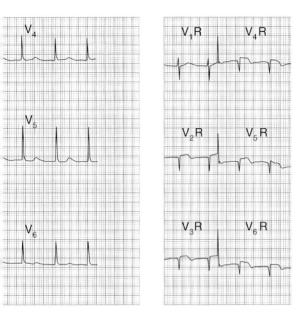

Fig. 4.12 Inferior and right ventricular infarction

Note
- Sinus rhythm
- Normal axis
- Raised ST segments in leads II, III, VF
- Raised ST segments in leads V_2R–V_5R
- Q waves in leads III, VF, V_2R–V_6R

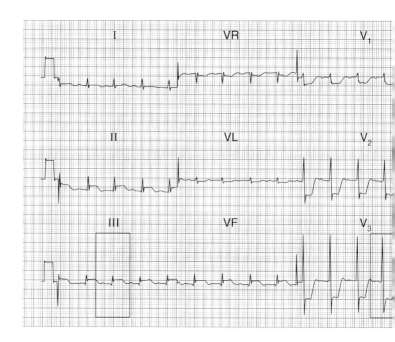

Multiple infarctions
Infarction of more than one part of the left ventricle causes
changes in several different ECG territories. This usually implies
disease in more than one of the main coronary arteries. The ECG
in Figure 4.13 shows an acute inferior myocardial infarction and
marked anterior ST segment depression. Later, coronary
angiography showed that this patient had a significant stenosis of
the left main coronary artery.

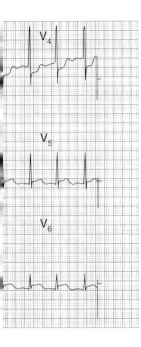

Fig. 4.13 Acute inferior infarction and anterior ischaemia

Note
- Sinus rhythm
- Normal axis
- Raised ST segments in leads II, III, VF
- ST depression in leads V_1–V_4

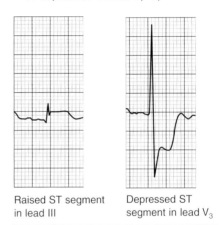

Raised ST segment in lead III

Depressed ST segment in lead V_3

Figure 4.14 is the record from a patient with an acute inferior myocardial infarction. Poor R wave progression in leads V_2–V_4 indicates an old anterior infarction.

Figure 4.15 is an ECG showing acute inferior infarction and anterior T wave inversion due to a 'non-Q wave' infarction (see p. 266).

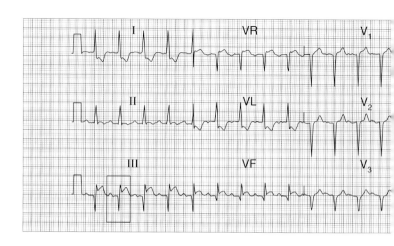

Fig. 4.15 Acute inferior infarction and anterior non-Q wave infarction

Note
- Sinus rhythm
- Normal axis
- Q waves in leads II, III, VF
- ST segment elevation in leads II, III, VF
- T wave inversion in leads V_3–V_5

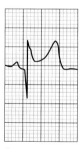

Q wave and ST segment elevation in lead III

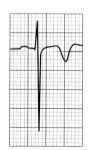

Inverted T wave in lead V_4

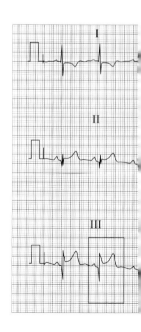

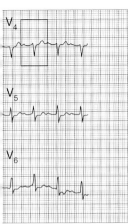

Fig. 4.14 Acute inferior and old anterior infarctions

Note
- Sinus rhythm
- Normal axis
- Q waves in leads III, VF
- Raised ST segments in leads III, VF
- Poor R wave progression in anterior leads

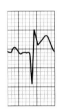

Q wave and raised
ST segment in lead III

Loss of R wave
in lead V₄

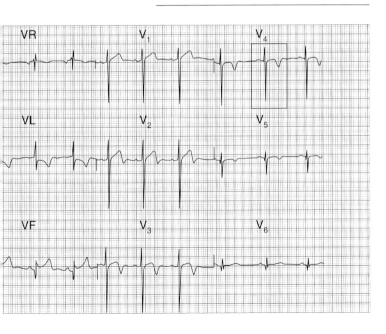

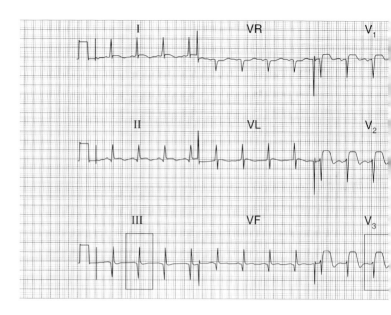

Figure 4.16 is an ECG showing an acute anterior myocardial infarction. Deep Q waves in leads III and VF indicate an old inferior infarction.

Bundle branch block and myocardial infarction
With left bundle branch block (LBBB) (Fig. 4.17) no changes due to myocardial infarction can be seen. However, this does not mean that the ECG can be totally disregarded. If a patient is admitted with chest pain that could be ischaemic and the ECG shows LBBB that is known to be new, it can be assumed that an acute infarction has occurred and appropriate treatment should be given.

Figure 4.18 is the record from another patient presenting with chest pain who had LBBB, but there are important differences from Figure 4.17. Peaked P waves suggest right atrial hypertrophy.

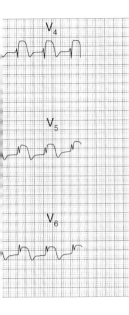

Fig. 4.16 Acute anterior and old inferior infarctions

Note
- Sinus rhythm
- Normal axis
- Q waves in leads II, III, VF
- ST segment elevation in leads V_2–V_6

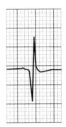

Q wave in lead III

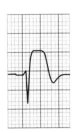

Raised ST segment in lead V_3

'Clockwise rotation' with no left ventricular QRS pattern in lead V_6 raises the possibility of either a pulmonary embolus (see p. 335) or chronic lung disease.

Right bundle branch block (RBBB) will not necessarily obscure the pattern of inferior infarction (Fig. 4.19).

Anterior infarction is more difficult to detect, but RBBB does not affect the ST segment and when this is raised in a patient who clinically has had an infarction, the change is probably significant (Fig. 4.20).

ST segment depression associated with RBBB does indicate ischaemia (Fig. 4.21).

However, T wave inversion in the anterior leads (Fig. 4.22) is more difficult to interpret because it is a common feature of RBBB itself.

259

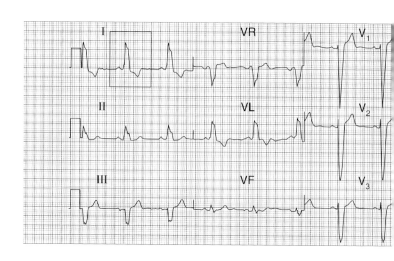

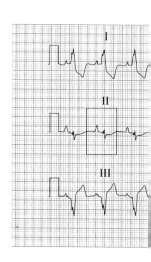

Fig. 4.18 Left bundle branch block, ?right ventricular overload

Note
- Sinus rhythm
- Peaked P waves in leads I, II
- LBBB pattern, most obvious in leads I, II
- Persistent S wave in lead V_6

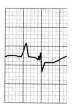

Peaked P wave in lead II

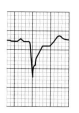

Persistent S wave in lead V_6

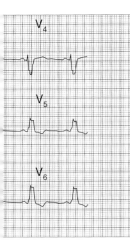

Fig. 4.17 Left bundle branch block

Note

- Sinus rhythm
- Normal axis
- Wide QRS complexes with LBBB pattern
- Inverted T waves in leads I, VL, V_5, V_6

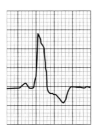

Broad QRS complex and inverted T wave in lead I

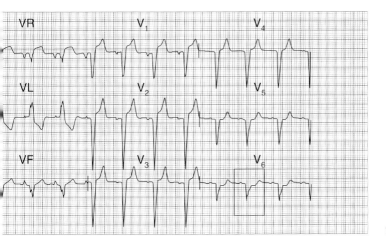

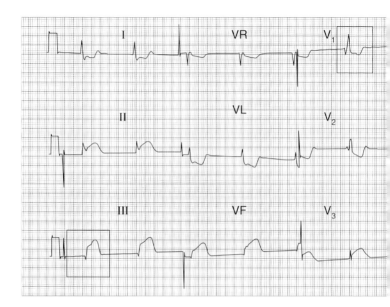

Fig. 4.20 Right bundle branch block and anterior infarction

Note
- Sinus rhythm
- Normal axis
- RBBB pattern
- Raised ST segments in leads V_2–V_4

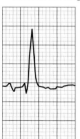

RSR^1 pattern in lead V_1

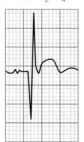

Raised ST segment in lead V_3

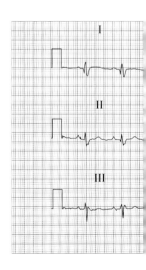

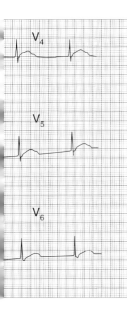

Fig. 4.19 Right bundle branch block and acute inferior infarction

Note
- Sinus rhythm
- Normal axis
- Wide QRS complex with RSR^1 pattern in lead V$_1$
- Raised ST segments in leads II, III, VF

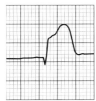

Raised ST segments in lead III

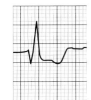

RSR^1 pattern in lead V$_1$

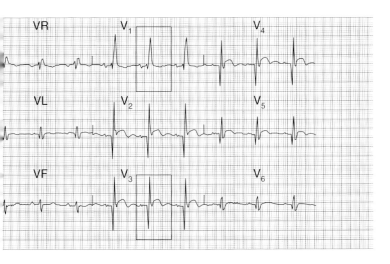

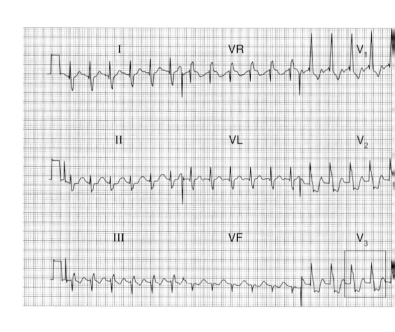

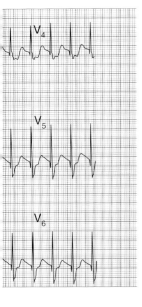

Fig. 4.21 Right bundle branch block and anterior ischaemia

Note
- Sinus rhythm
- RBBB pattern
- ST segment depression in leads V_2–V_4

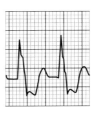

ST segment depression in lead V_3

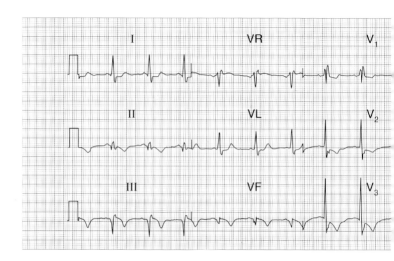

Non-Q wave infarction
When the infarction does not involve the whole thickness of the
ventricular wall, no electrical 'window' will be formed so there
will be no Q waves. There will, however, be an abnormality of
repolarization that leads to T wave inversion. This pattern is most
commonly seen in the anterior and lateral leads (Fig. 4.23). This
ECG pattern is sometimes called 'subendocardial infarction', but
the pathological changes seen in heart muscle after myocardial
infarction often do not fit neatly into 'subendocardial' or 'full
thickness' patterns. Acute non-Q wave infarction is usually
associated with a rise in the blood troponin level. Compared
to patients with Q wave infarctions, those with non-Q wave
infarctions have a high incidence of reinfarction during the
following 3 months, but thereafter their fatality rates are similar.

Ischaemia
Cardiac ischaemia causes horizontal ST segment depression.
This appears and disappears with the pain of stable angina, but

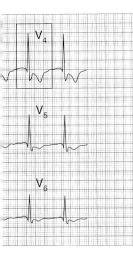

Fig. 4.22 Inferior infarction, right bundle branch block, ?anterior ischaemia

Note
- Sinus rhythm
- Q waves with inverted T waves in leads II, III, VF
- RBBB pattern
- Deep T wave inversion in leads V₃–V₄

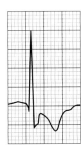

T wave inversion in lead V₄

persistent pain and ST segment depression (Fig. 4.24) may be associated with a rise in troponin level. When this occurs the prognosis is essentially the same as following a non-Q wave infarction.

If a patient has chest pain that persists long enough for him or her to seek hospital admission, and the ECG shows ST segment depression, the outlook is relatively poor – even when the ST segment depression is not marked (Figs 4.25 and 4.26) and there is no rise in troponin level. These patients usually need further investigation, though on the whole they can be managed as outpatients.

Ischaemia may be precipitated by an arrhythmia, and will resolve when either the heart rate is controlled or the arrhythmia is corrected. The ECG in Figure 4.27 shows ischaemia during atrial fibrillation with a rapid ventricular rate (this patient had not been treated with digoxin). The ECG in Figure 4.28 shows ischaemic ST segment depression in a patient with an AV nodal tachycardia and a ventricular rate of over 200/min.

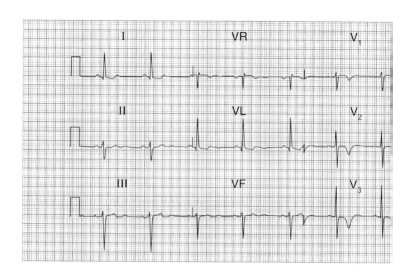

Fig. 4.24 **Anterior ischaemia, possible old inferior infarction**

Note
- Sinus rhythm
- Normal axis
- Small Q waves in leads III, VF
- Inverted T waves in lead III
- Marked ST segment depression in leads V_2–V_6

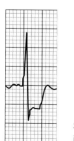

ST segment depression in lead V_4

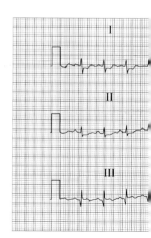

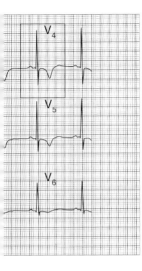

Fig. 4.23 Anterior non-Q wave infarction

Note
- Sinus rhythm
- Left axis deviation
- Normal QRS complexes
- Inverted T waves in all chest leads

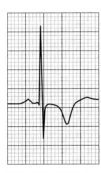

Inverted T wave in lead V_4

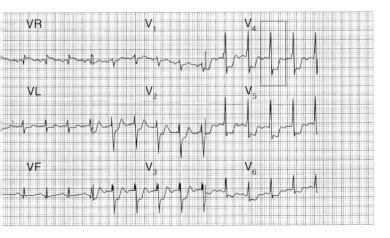

269

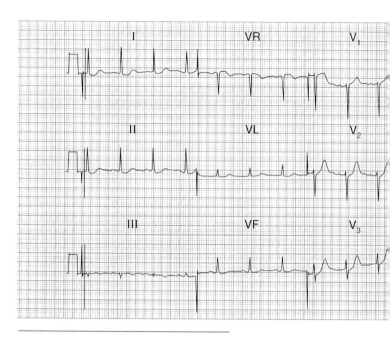

Fig. 4.26 Anterolateral ischaemia

Note

- Sinus rhythm
- Possible left atrial hypertrophy (bifid P wave in lead I)
- Normal axis
- Normal QRS complexes
- ST segment depression in leads I, II, V_4–V_6

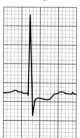

ST segment depression in lead V_5

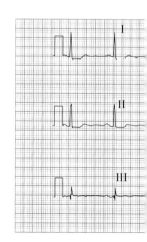

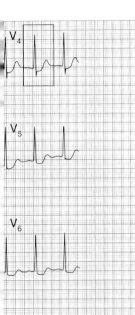

Fig. 4.25 Anterior ischaemia

Note
- Sinus rhythm
- Normal axis
- Normal QRS complexes
- ST segment depression in leads V_4–V_6

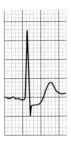

ST segment depression in lead V_4

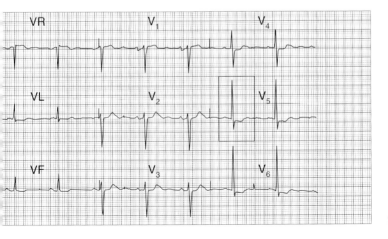

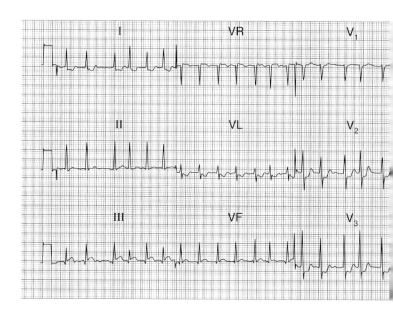

Fig. 4.28 Junctional tachycardia with anterior ischaemia

Note
- Regular narrow complex tachycardia rate 200/min
- No P waves
- ST segment depression in leads V_2–V_6

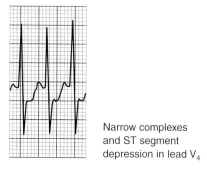

Narrow complexes and ST segment depression in lead V_4

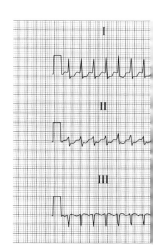

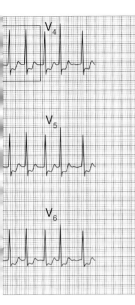

Fig. 4.27 Atrial fibrillation and anterior ischaemia

Note
- Atrial fibrillation, ventricular rate about 130/min
- Normal axis
- Normal QRS complexes
- ST segment depression in leads V_2–V_6

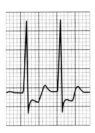

ST segment depression in lead V_4

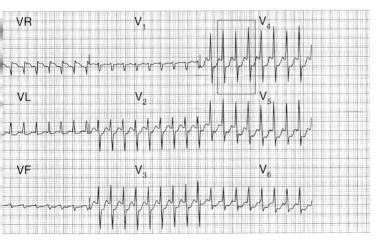

273

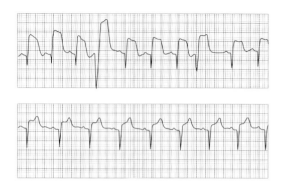

Fig. 4.29 Prinzmetal's variant angina

Note
- The two strips form a continuous record
- Initially the patient had pain and the ST segment was raised
- The fourth beat is probably a ventricular extrasystole
- As the patient's pain settled the ST segment returned to normal

Prinzmetal's 'variant' angina
Angina can occur at rest due to spasm of the coronary arteries. This is accompanied by elevation rather than depression of the ST segments. The ECG appearance is similar to that of an acute myocardial infarction, but the ST segment returns to normal as the pain settles (Fig. 4.29). This ECG appearance was first described by Prinzmetal, and it is sometimes called 'variant' angina.

Exercise testing
Although any form of exercise that induces pain should produce ischaemic changes in the ECG, it is best to use a reproducible test that patients find reasonably easy to perform, and to use carefully graded increments of exercise. The use of nonstandard tests means that the results may be difficult to interpret, and that repeated tests in the same patient cannot be compared meaningfully. It is important to remember that exercise testing provides much useful

information in addition to causing changes in the ST segment of the ECG. Things to look for during an exercise test include:

- The patient's attitude to exercise
- The reasons for exercise limitation:
  - chest pain
  - breathlessness
  - claudication
  - fatigue
  - musculoskeletal problems
- The pumping capability of the heart
  - maximum heart rate achieved
  - maximum rise in blood pressure
- Physical fitness
  - workload at which maximum heart rate is achieved
  - duration of tachycardia following exercise
- Ischaemic changes in the ECG
- Exercise-induced arrhythmias.

Reproducible exercise testing needs either a bicycle ergometer or a treadmill. In either case, the exercise should begin at a low level that the patient finds easy, and should be made progressively more difficult. On a bicycle, the pedal speed should be kept constant and the workload increased in 25 watt steps. On a treadmill, both the slope and the speed can be changed and the protocol evolved by Bruce (Table 4.1) is the one most commonly used.

Alternatively, a Naughton protocol can be used: this involves a much slower increase of workload (Table 4.2).

Table 4.1 Bruce protocol for exercise testing using a treadmill, 3 min at each stage

	Low level			Ordinary level				
Stage	01	02	03	1	2	3	4	5
Speed (km/h)	2.7	2.7	2.7	2.7	4.0	5.5	6.8	8.0
Slope (degrees)	0	1.3	2.6	4.3	5.4	6.3	7.2	8.1

Table 4.2 Modified Naughton protocol, 2 min at each stage

Stage	0	1	2	3	4	5	6	7	8	9	10
Speed (km/h)	1.6	2.4	3.2	3.2	3.2	4.8	4.8	4.8	4.8	5.5	5.5
Slope (degrees)	0	0	2	4	6	4.3	5.7	7.1	8.5	8	9

A 12-lead ECG, the heart rate and the blood pressure should be recorded at the end of each exercise period. The maximum heart rate and blood pressure are in some ways more important than the maximum workload achieved, because the latter is markedly influenced by physical fitness.

Indications for discontinuing the test are:

1. At the request of the patient, because of pain, breathlessness, fatigue or dizziness.
2. If the systolic blood pressure begins to fall. Normally, systolic pressure will rise progressively with increasing exercise level, but in any subject a point will be reached at which systolic pressure reaches a plateau and then starts to fall. A fall of 10 mmHg is an indication that the heart is not pumping effectively and the test should be stopped; if it is continued, the patient will become dizzy and may fall. In healthy subjects, a fall in systolic pressure is seen only at high workloads, but in patients with severe heart disease the systolic pressure may fail to rise on exercise. The amount of exercise the patient can carry out before the systolic pressure falls is thus a useful indicator of the severity of any heart disease.
3. It is conventional to discontinue the test if the heart rate increases to 80% of the predicted maximum for the patient's age: this maximum can be calculated in beats/min by subtracting the patient's age in years from 220. Patients with severe heart disease will usually fail to attain 80% of their predicted maximum heart rate, and the peak rate is another useful indicator of the state of the patient's heart. It is, of course, important to take note of any treatment the patient may be receiving, because a beta-blocker will prevent the normal increase in heart rate.

4. Exercise should be discontinued immediately if an arrhythmia occurs. The use of exercise testing to provoke arrhythmias is discussed in Chapter 3. Many patients will have ventricular extrasystoles during exercise. These can be ignored unless their frequency begins to rise, or a couplet of extrasystoles occurs.

5. The test should be stopped if the ST segment in any lead becomes depressed by 4 mm. 2 mm of horizontal depression in any lead is usually taken as indicating that a diagnosis of ischaemia can be made (a 'positive' test), and if the aim of the test is to confirm or refute a diagnosis of angina there is no point in continuing once this has occurred. It may, however, be useful to find out just how much a patient can do, and if this is the aim of the test it is not unreasonable to continue, if the patient's symptoms are not severe.

The final report of the test should indicate the duration of exercise, the workload achieved, the maximum heart rate and systolic pressure, the reason for discontinuing the test, and a description of any arrhythmias or ST segment changes.

An exercise test is usually considered 'positive' for ischaemia if horizontal ST segment depression of 2 mm or more develops during exercise, and resolves on resting. A diagnosis of ischaemia becomes almost certain if these changes are accompanied by the appearance and then disappearance of angina. Figures 4.30 and 4.31 show an ECG that was normal when the patient was at rest, but which demonstrated clear ischaemia during exercise.

There are, however, other ECG changes that may be seen during an exercise test. Figures 4.32 and 4.33 show the records of tests in a patient who had had an anterior myocardial infarction some weeks previously. At rest, some ST segment elevation persisted in the anterior leads. During exercise the ST elevation became more marked. The reasons for this are uncertain. It has been suggested that the change is due to the development of an abnormality of left ventricular contraction, but other evidence suggests that it is simply another ECG manifestation of ischaemia. There is, however, no doubt that this is an abnormal result.

When the ST segment becomes depressed during exercise, but slopes upwards, the change is not an indication of ischaemia (Figs 4.34 and 4.35). Deciding whether ST segment depression slopes upwards or is horizontal can be quite difficult.

277

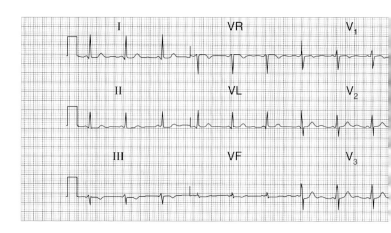

Fig. 4.31 **Exercise-induced ischaemia**

Note
- Same patient as in Figure 4.30
- Sinus rhythm, 138/min
- Horizontal ST segment depression in leads II, III, VF, V_4–V_6

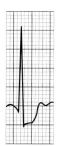

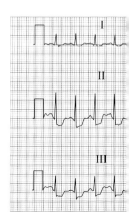

Horizontal ST segment depression in lead V_5

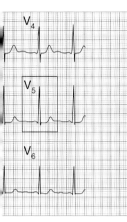

Fig. 4.30 Probably normal record

Note
- Sinus rhythm
- Normal axis
- Normal QRS complexes
- Some nonspecific T wave change in leads III, VF

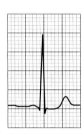

Normal ST segment in lead V_5

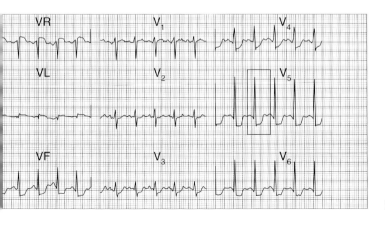

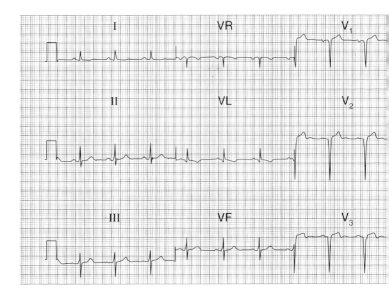

Fig. 4.33 Exercise-induced ST segment elevation

Note
- Same patient as in Figure 4.32
- Compared with Figure 4.32, the ST segments are higher in leads V_3, V_4

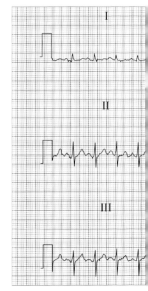

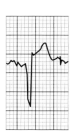

More ST segment elevation in lead V_4

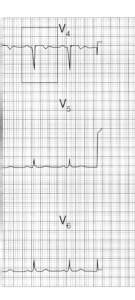

Fig. 4.32 Anterior infarction, ?age

Note
- Sinus rhythm
- Normal axis
- Q waves in leads V_2–V_4
- Slight ST segment elevation in leads V_2–V_4

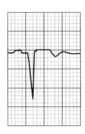

Q wave, slight ST segment elevation and inverted T wave in lead V_4

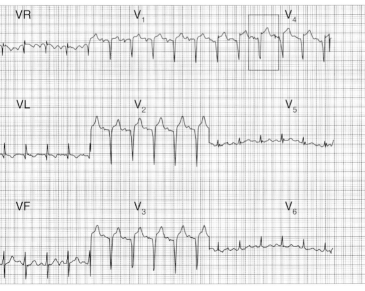

281

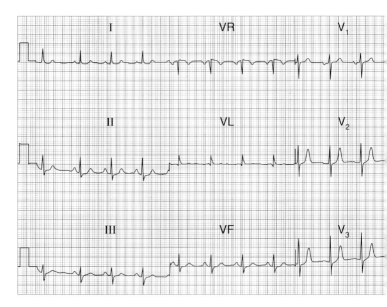

Fig. 4.35 Exercise-induced ST segment depression

Note

- Same patient as Figure 4.34
- On exercise there is ST segment depression which slopes upwards
- This is not diagnostic of ischaemia but the change in lead V$_5$ is suspicious

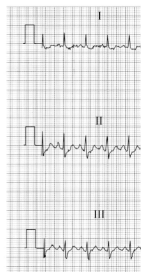

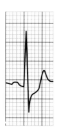

Upward-sloping ST segment depression in lead V$_4$

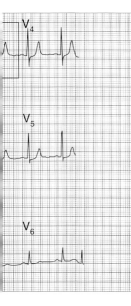

Fig. 4.34 Normal ECG

Note
- Sinus rhythm
- Normal axis
- Normal QRS complexes
- Possible minimal ST segment depression in lead V_5

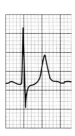

Normal ST segment in lead V_4

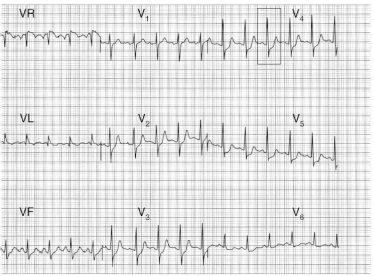

'False positive' changes also occur when exercise testing is performed in patients taking digoxin. Figures 4.36 and 4.37 show the results of an exercise test in a patient being treated with digoxin, whose coronary angiogram was normal.

In a patient suspected of having coronary disease, exercise testing gives the 'right' answer perhaps 80% of the time. All tests at times give 'false positive' and 'false negative' results, reflecting their sensitivity and specificity. In an asymptomatic subject in whom the likelihood of coronary disease is low, the chance of a 'false positive' result may be higher than the chance of a 'true positive'. The greater the likelihood that the patient has coronary disease, the

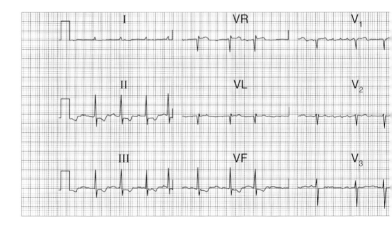

more likely it is that a positive test is 'true' rather than 'false'. The statistics (Bayes' theorem) may seem complex, but the important thing is to remember that exercise testing is not infallible.

Exercise testing thus has to be used and interpreted with care. Remember also that it is not without risk. The ECGs in Figures 4.38, 4.39 and 4.40 are from a patient whose resting ECG was normal, but he began to develop ventricular extrasystoles as the test proceeded and then suddenly developed ventricular fibrillation. This occurs in about 1 in 10 000 tests, which shows the need for full resuscitation facilities to be available at the time of exercise testing.

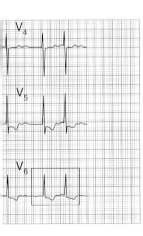

Fig. 4.36 Atrial fibrillation: digoxin effect at rest

Note
- Atrial fibrillation
- ST segments slope downwards and T waves are inverted in leads V_5, V_6: typical of digoxin effect

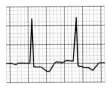

Downward-sloping ST segment and inverted T wave in lead V_6

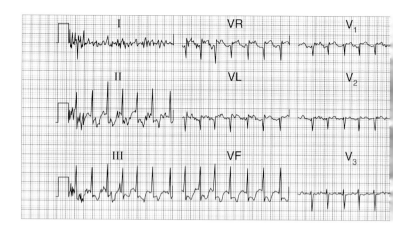

Fig. 4.38 Pre-exercise: normal ECG

Note
- Sinus rhythm
- Heart rate 75/min
- Possible nonspecific ST segment depression in lead V_6

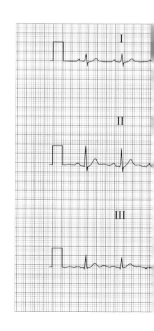

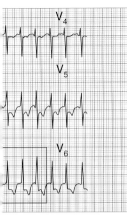

Fig. 4.37 Atrial fibrillation: digoxin effect on exercise

Note
- Same patient as Figure 4.36
- Heart rate 165/min
- ST segment depression in lead V6 could be ischaemic but could be a 'false positive' due to digoxin

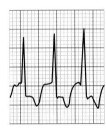

Further ST segment depression in lead V_6

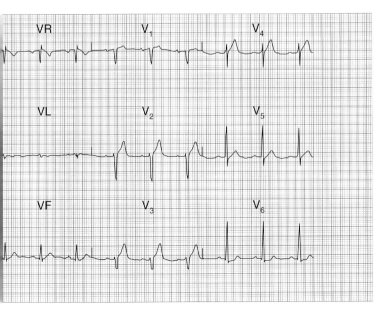

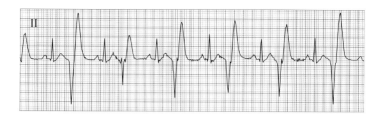

Fig. 4.39 Exercise-induced ventricular extrasystoles

Note
- Same patient as in Figures 4.38 and 4.40
- Sinus rhythm with coupled ventricular extrasystoles

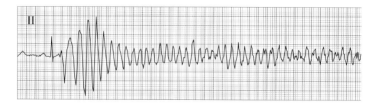

Fig. 4.40 Exercise-induced ventricular fibrillation

Note
- Same patient as in Figures 4.38 and 4.39
- One sinus beat is followed by an extrasystole with the R on T phenomenon
- A few beats of ventricular tachycardia decay into ventricular fibrillation

The ECG in pulmonary embolism

Most patients with a pulmonary embolus will have sinus tachycardia, but otherwise a normal ECG.

The ECG abnormalities that may occur in pulmonary embolism are those associated with right ventricular problems:

- Right axis deviation
- Dominant R wave in lead V_1
- Inverted T waves in leads V_1–V_3, and sometimes V_4
- RBBB pattern
- Q wave and inverted T wave in lead III.

Supraventricular arrhythmias, especially atrial fibrillation, may also occur. There is no particular sequence in which these changes develop, and they can be seen in any combination. The full ECG pattern of right ventricular hypertrophy (right axis deviation, dominant R waves in lead V_1, inverted T waves in leads V_1–V_4, and persistent S waves in lead V_6) is usually only seen in patients with long-standing thromboembolic pulmonary hypertension.

Figures 4.41, 4.42, 4.43 and 4.44 show the records from four patients with a pulmonary embolus – but remember, in most patients the ECG is normal.

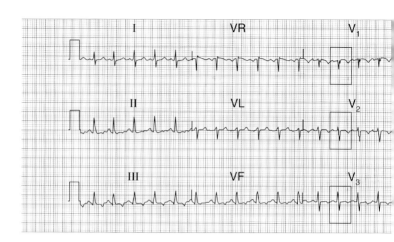

Fig. 4.42 Pulmonary embolus

Note
- Sinus rhythm
- Right axis deviation
- Persistent S wave in lead V_6
- T wave inversion in leads V_1–V_4

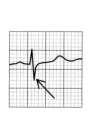

Persistent S wave
in lead V_6

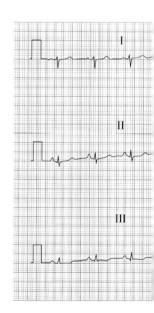

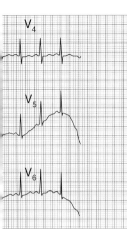

Fig. 4.41 Pulmonary embolus

Note
- Sinus rhythm, 130/min
- Normal axis
- Normal QRS complexes
- Inverted T wave in leads V_1–V_3, VF

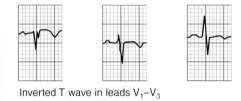

Inverted T wave in leads V_1–V_3

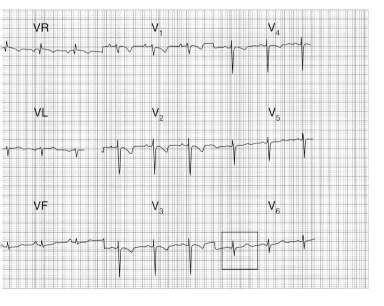

291

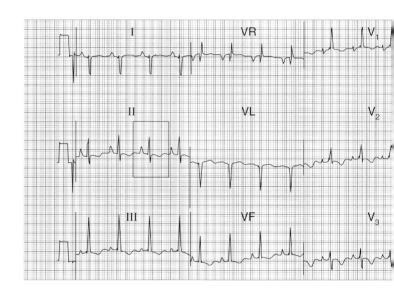

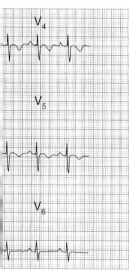

Fig. 4.43 Pulmonary embolus

Note
- Sinus rhythm
- Peaked P wave suggests right atrial hypertrophy
- Right axis deviation
- RBBB pattern
- Persistent S wave in lead V_6

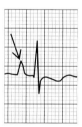

Peaked P wave in lead II

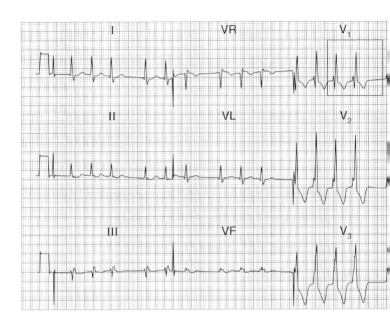

The ECG in other causes of chest pain

Pericarditis

Pericarditis classically causes raised ST segments in most leads
(Fig. 4.45). This may suggest a widespread acute infarction, but
in pericarditis the ST segment remains elevated and Q waves do
not develop. This pattern is actually very rare: most patients with
pericarditis have either a normal ECG, or a variety of nonspecific
ST segment/T wave changes.

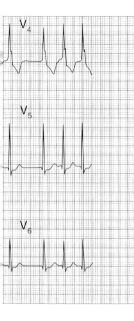

Fig. 4.44 Pulmonary embolus

Note
- Atrial fibrillation
- RBBB pattern

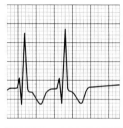

RSR^1 pattern in lead V$_1$

Aortic stenosis

Aortic stenosis is an important cause of angina. The ECG should show left ventricular hypertrophy (Fig. 4.46) – however, the ECG is an unreliable guide to left ventricular hypertrophy (see Ch. 5). The difficulty of distinguishing this from ischaemia is also discussed in Chapter 5.

The presence of left ventricular hypertrophy in the ECG of a patient with chest pain also raises the possibility of aortic dissection.

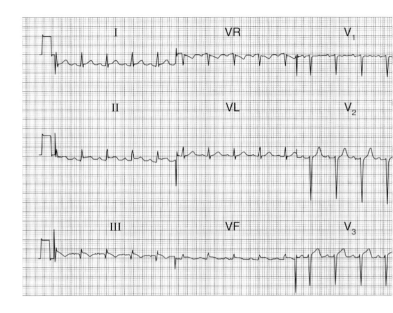

Fig. 4.46 Left ventricular hypertrophy

Note
- Sinus rhythm
- Tall R waves in leads V_5, V_6
- Inverted T waves in lateral leads

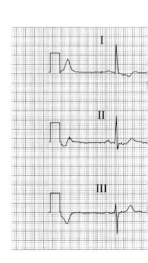

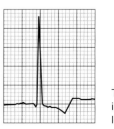

Tall R wave and inverted T wave in lead V_6

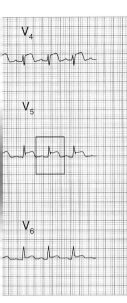

Fig. 4.45 Pericarditis

Note
- Sinus rhythm
- Normal axis
- Normal QRS complexes
- ST segment elevation in leads I, II, III, VF, V_3–V_6

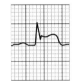

ST segment elevation in lead V_5

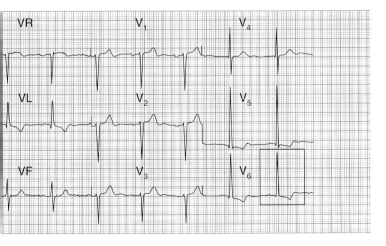

ECG pitfalls in the diagnosis of ischaemia

The normal variants of the ECG have been described in Chapter 2. The important ones that may be confused with ischaemia are:

- Septal Q waves (mainly in leads II, VL, V_6)
- Q waves in lead III but not VF
- Anterior T wave inversion (not uncommon in lead V_2, common in black people in leads V_2, V_3 and sometimes V_4)
- 'High take-off' ST segments.

Several abnormal ECG patterns may cause difficulty in making a diagnosis in patients with chest pain, which was the presenting problem in the following examples.

The ECG in Figure 4.47 shows a dominant R wave in lead V_1. This might be due to right ventricular hypertrophy or to a posterior infarction. Occasionally it could be a normal variant. Here, the normal axis goes against a diagnosis of right ventricular hypertrophy. In this case, a review of previous ECGs from the patient showed that the dominant R wave was due to a posterior infarction.

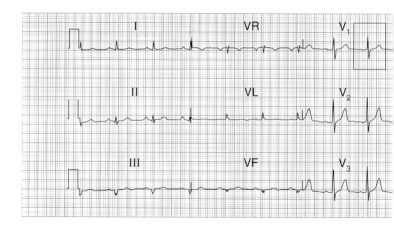

The ECG in Figure 4.48 also shows a dominant R wave in lead V_1. In a patient with chest pain, a posterior infarction might again be considered. However, the PR interval is short and there is a delta wave, so this shows a Wolff–Parkinson–White (WPW) syndrome.

It is, however, repolarization (T wave) changes that cause most problems. The lateral T wave inversion in the ECG in Figure 4.49 might suggest ischaemia, but again this is a WPW syndrome, in which repolarization abnormalities are common.

The anterior and lateral T wave inversion in the ECG in Figure 4.50 suggests either a non-Q wave infarction or hypertrophic cardiomyopathy. This particular patient was white, asymptomatic and had no family history of arrhythmias or any cardiac disease. There was no echocardiographic evidence of cardiomyopathy, and coronary angiography was normal. The ECG reverted to normal on exercise, and the T wave inversion remained unexplained.

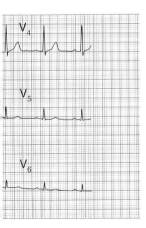

Fig. 4.47 Old posterior infarction

Note
- Sinus rhythm
- Normal axis
- Dominant R waves in leads V_1, V_2
- No other abnormalities

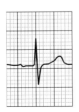

Dominant R wave in lead V_1

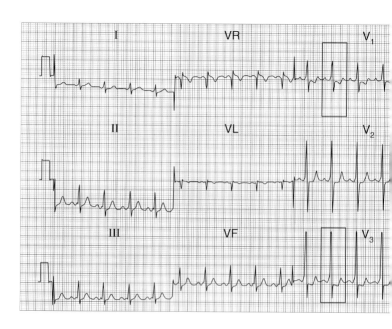

Fig. 4.49 Wolff–Parkinson–White syndrome

Note
- Sinus rhythm
- Short PR interval
- Left axis deviation
- Delta wave
- Inverted T waves in leads I, VL, V_5, V_6
- No dominant R wave in lead V_1: WPW syndrome type B

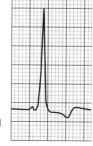

Short PR interval and delta wave in lead VL

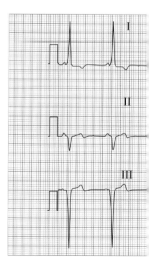

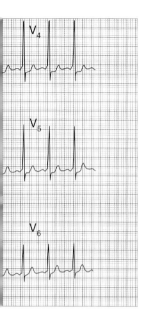

Fig. 4.48 Wolff–Parkinson–White syndrome

Note
- Sinus rhythm
- Short PR interval
- Slurred upstroke to QRS complexes
- Dominant R wave in lead V_1: WPW syndrome type A

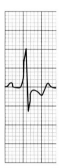

Dominant R wave in lead V_1

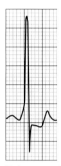

Delta wave in lead V_3

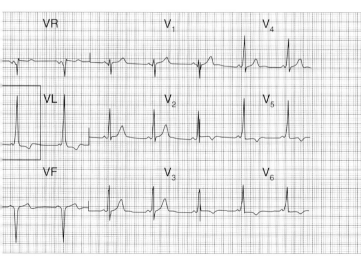

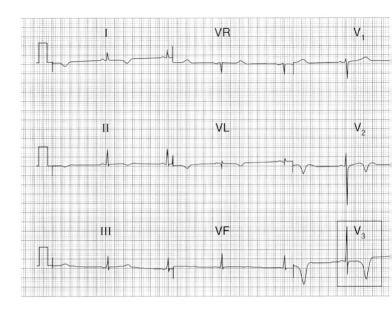

Differentiation between lateral ischaemia and left ventricular hypertrophy on the ECG is extremely difficult. The ECG in Figure 4.51 shows lateral T wave inversion. There are small Q waves in leads III and VF, suggesting a possible old inferior infarction, and the QRS complexes in the chest leads are not particularly tall. Nevertheless, in this patient the lateral T wave inversion was due to left ventricular hypertrophy.

The patient whose ECG is shown in Figure 4.52 had mild hypertension. The QRS complexes are tall (see Ch. 5) and there is lateral T wave inversion, suggesting left ventricular hypertrophy. However, there is also T wave inversion in leads V_3 and V_4, which is unusual in left ventricular hypertrophy. This patient had severe narrowing of the left main coronary artery.

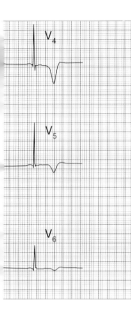

Fig. 4.50 Unexplained T wave abnormality

Note
- Sinus rhythm
- Normal axis
- Normal QRS complexes
- QT interval 600 ms
- T wave inversion in leads I, II, VL, V_2–V_6

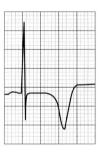

Long QT interval and inverted T wave in lead V_3

Digoxin therapy causes downward-sloping ST segment depression and T wave inversion (see Ch. 6), particularly in the lateral leads, as is seen in Figure 4.53. The fact that the rhythm is atrial fibrillation with a controlled ventricular rate suggests that the patient is being treated with digoxin. However, T wave inversion in leads V_3 and V_4 is much more likely to be due to ischaemia, as was the case here.

An extremely common finding on the ECG is 'nonspecific T wave flattening' (Fig. 4.54). When a patient is completely well and the heart is clinically normal, this is of no importance. However, in a patient with chest pain that appears to be cardiac, 'nonspecific' ST segment/T wave changes may indicate ischaemia.

Table 4.3 summarizes some of the potential pitfalls in the diagnosis of the cause of chest pain.

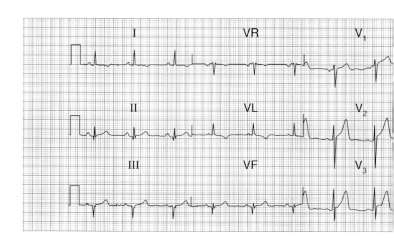

Fig. 4.52 Old anterolateral non-Q wave infarction

Note
- Sinus rhythm
- Normal axis
- Tall QRS complexes
- T wave inversion in leads I, VL, V_3–V_6, but this is more marked in lead V_4 than in V_6

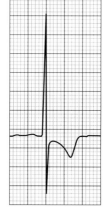

Inverted T wave in lead V_4

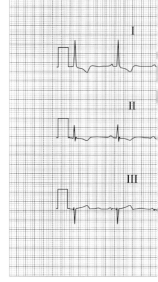

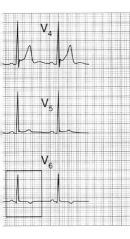

Fig. 4.51 Left ventricular hypertrophy

Note
- Sinus rhythm
- Normal axis
- Height of R wave in lead V_5 + depth of S wave in lead V_2 = 37 mm
- High take-off ST segment in lead V_4
- T wave inversion in leads I, VL, V_6

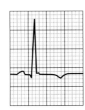

Inverted T wave in lead V_6

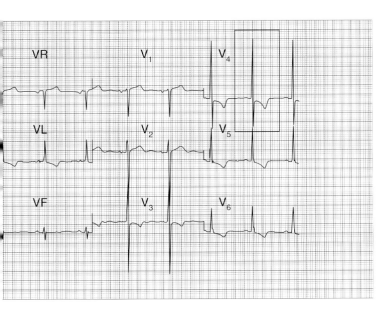

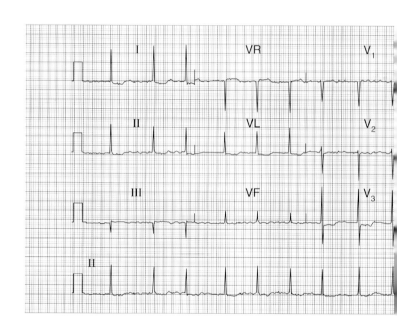

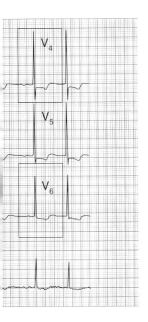

Fig. 4.53 Digoxin effect and ischaemia

Note
- Atrial fibrillation
- Normal axis
- Normal QRS complexes
- Horizontal ST segment in lead V$_4$
- Downward-sloping ST segment in lead V$_6$
- Inverted T waves in leads V$_3$, V$_4$

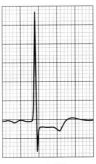

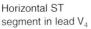

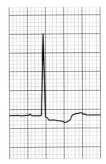

Horizontal ST segment in lead V$_4$

Downward-sloping ST segment in lead V$_6$

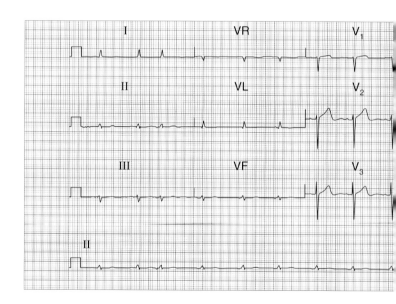

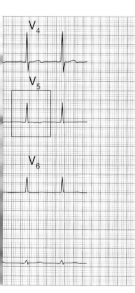

Fig. 4.54 Nonspecific T wave flattening

Note
- Recorded at half sensitivity
- Sinus rhythm with supraventricular extrasystoles
- Normal QRS complexes
- Flat T waves in leads I, VL, V_5, V_6

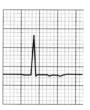

Flat T wave in lead V_5

Table 4.3 ECG pitfalls in the diagnosis of chest pain

Condition	ECG pattern	May be confused with
Normal record	Q waves in lead III but not VF	Inferior infarction
	T wave inversion in leads V_1–V_3 (especially in black people)	Anterior infarction
Left ventricular hypertrophy	T wave inversion in lateral leads	Ischaemia
Right ventricular hypertrophy	Dominant R waves in lead V_1	Posterior infarction
	Inverted T waves in leads V_1–V_3	Anterior infarction
Wolff–Parkinson–White syndrome	Inverted T waves in leads V_2–V_5	Anterior infarction
Hypertrophic cardiomyopathy	T wave inversion in leads V_2–V_5	Anterior infarction
Subarachnoid haemorrhage	T wave inversion in any leads	Ischaemia
Digoxin effect	Downward-sloping ST segment depression or T wave inversion, especially in leads V_5–V_6	Ischaemia

WHAT TO DO

It is essential to remember that while the ECG can on occasions be extremely helpful in the diagnosis of chest pain, frequently it is not. The history, and to a lesser extent the physical examination, are far more important.

Acute chest pain suggesting myocardial infarction

If the history suggests that the patient has had a myocardial infarction, the aims of treatment are:

1. Pain relief
2. Getting the patient quickly to an ambulance or hospital, where cardiac arrest can be properly managed should it occur
3. Making a more certain diagnosis
4. Instituting thrombolytic therapy, if there are no contraindications.

To reduce the risk of treating patients inappropriately, it is customary to give thrombolytic treatment only to those whose ECG shows changes that are at least suggestive of an infarction. These changes are any of the following:

- ST segment elevation ≥ 1 mm in two or more limb leads, or ≥ 2 mm in two or more chest leads
- LBBB, unless this is known to be of long standing.

Thrombolytic therapy is effective whichever site of infarction is indicated by the ECG. Right ventricular infarcts are treated in the same way as are left ventricular infarcts, except that vasodilators must be avoided in the treatment of right ventricular infarction – the left ventricle is often under-filled, and the administration of fluid (preferably with haemodynamic monitoring using a Swan–Ganz catheter) may be needed.

Old or equivocal ECG changes, or bundle branch block, do not provide sufficient indication for thrombolysis unless supported by measurements of cardiac enzyme levels.

The best-established thrombolytic regimen is:

- Soluble aspirin 300 mg, chewed immediately
- Streptokinase 1.5 m units, infused over 1.5 h
- Heparin i.v. for 24 h.

The alternative thrombolytic agents rt-PA (alteplase) or RPA (reteplase) may possibly cause less adverse reactions than streptokinase, but these are seldom severe with any agent, and may not justify the higher cost. They are indicated in patients who have previously been treated with streptokinase, and in whom the presence of antibodies may make streptokinase less effective and may increase the risk of severe allergic reaction.

There is no evidence that the routine use of prophylactic antiarrhythmic drugs is beneficial, and indeed it may be harmful.

Investigations for acute chest pain

Chest X-rays are seldom helpful and unless a pneumothorax or some other cause of pleurisy, or a dissecting aneurysm, seem possible the patient should not be detained in the A & E department waiting for an X-ray examination. Chest X-rays taken using portable equipment are seldom helpful.

Echocardiography is the investigation of choice if pericarditis is suspected, as most patients will have a pericardial effusion which is easily detected. Echocardiography may help in the diagnosis of an aortic dissection, but not reliably; CT scanning is probably the investigation of choice in such cases.

Investigations for chronic chest pain

Chronic or intermittent chest pain must be investigated and treated as the history dictates. If angina seems likely but the resting ECG is normal, an exercise test may be useful in establishing the diagnosis and giving a rough indication of the severity of the angina.

Coronary angiography is essential if coronary artery bypass grafting or percutaneous transluminal coronary angioplasty is being considered, so patients still symptomatic despite maximum medical therapy need to be investigated. Angiography is also necessary in young people with a strongly positive exercise test at a low workload (say, 3 mm depression at Bruce Stage 2 or less).

A trial of sublingual glyceryl trinitrate 0.5 mg may help make the diagnosis of angina, and in such cases patients should then be encouraged to use the drug liberally and prophylactically. Beta-blockers are the first-line agents for preventing angina. All have much the same effect, and a cardioselective agent such as atenolol 50–1000 mg daily is best. If the patient is unable to take a beta-blocker (e.g. because of asthma), treatment should start with a calcium-channel blocker such as amlodipine 5–10 mg. Beta-blockers and calcium-channel blockers can be combined, or a long-acting nitrate such as isosorbide mononitrate 20 mg twice daily can be substituted. The combination of two of these drug classes is sometimes helpful; the addition of the third seldom

provides much further benefit.

5
The ECG in patients with breathlessness

HISTORY AND EXAMINATION

There are many causes of breathlessness (see Table 5.1). Everyone is breathless at times, and people who are physically unfit or who are overweight will be more breathless than others. Breathlessness can also result from anxiety, but when it is due to physical illness the important causes are anaemia, heart disease and lung disease; a combination of causes is common. The most important function of the history is to help to determine whether the patient does indeed have a physical illness and if so, which system is affected.

Breathlessness in heart disease is due either to increased lung stiffness as a result of pulmonary congestion, or to pulmonary oedema. Pulmonary congestion occurs when the left atrial pressure is high. A high left atrial pressure occurs either in mitral

Table 5.1 Causes of breathlessness

Cause	Underlying cause
Physiological and psychological	Lack of fitness
	Obesity
	Pregnancy
	Locomotor diseases (including ankylosing spondylitis)
	Anxiety
Heart disease	
Left ventricular failure	Ischaemia
	Mitral regurgitation
	Aortic stenosis
	Aortic regurgitation
	Congenital disease
	Cardiomyopathy
	Arrhythmias
High left atrial pressure	Mitral stenosis
	Atrial myxoma
Lung disease	Any interstitial lung disease (e.g. infection, tumour, infiltration)
	Pulmonary embolism
	Pleural effusion
	Pneumothorax
Pericardial disease	Constrictive pericarditis
Anaemia	

stenosis or in left ventricular failure. Pulmonary oedema occurs when the left atrial pressure exceeds the oncotic pressure exerted by the plasma proteins.

Congestive cardiac failure (right heart failure secondary to left heart failure) can be difficult to distinguish from cor pulmonale (right heart failure due to lung disease) With both, the patient is breathless. Both are associated with pulmonary crackles – in left heart failure due to pulmonary oedema, and in cor pulmonale due to the lung disease. Also in both, the patient may complain of orthopnoea. In heart failure, this is due to the return to the effective circulation of blood that was pooled in the legs. In patients with chest disease (especially chronic obstructive airways disease) orthopnoea results from a need to use diaphragmatic respiration. Both pulmonary congestion and lung disease can cause a diffuse wheeze. The diagnosis therefore depends on a positive identification, either in the history or on examination, of heart or lung disease.

The main value of the ECG in patients with breathlessness is to indicate whether heart disease of any sort is present, and whether the left or the right side of the heart is affected. The ECG is best at identifying rhythm abnormalities (which may lead to left ventricular impairment and so to breathlessness) and conditions affecting the left ventricle – particularly ischaemia. The patient with a completely normal ECG is unlikely to have left ventricular failure, though of course there are exceptions. Lung disease eventually affects the right side of the heart, and may cause changes suggesting that significant lung disease is present. Thus as well as suggesting a pathological cause of breathlessness the ECG can, by showing which part of the heart is affected, help with the diagnosis.

RHYTHM PROBLEMS

A sudden rhythm change is a common cause of breathlessness, and even of frank pulmonary oedema. Arrhythmias can be paroxysmal, so the patient may be in sinus rhythm when examined. A patient who is suddenly breathless may not be aware of an arrhythmia. When sudden breathlessness is associated with palpitations it is important to establish whether the breathlessness or the palpitations came first – palpitations following breathlessness may be due to the sinus tachycardia of anxiety. The ECG in Figure 5.1 is from a patient who developed pulmonary oedema due to the onset of uncontrolled atrial fibrillation.

Less dramatic rhythm abnormalities can also contribute to breathlessness, especially to breathlessness on exertion. This is true of both fast and slow rhythms. The ECG in Figure 5.2 is from a patient who was breathless on exercise, partly because of coupled ventricular extrasystoles, which markedly reduced cardiac output as a result of an effective rate of half of the 76/min recorded on the ECG. **315**

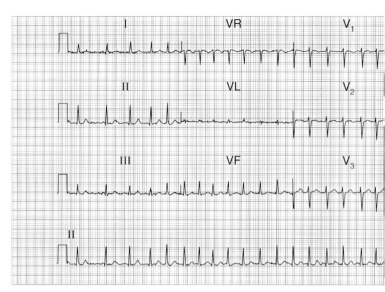

Fig. 5.2 Atrial fibrillation with coupled ventricular extrasystoles

Note

- Atrial fibrillation, with slow and regular ventricular response
- Coupled ventricular extrasystoles
- In supraventricular beats, V_5 and V_6 show a deep wide S wave, suggesting RBBB
- ?Digoxin toxicity

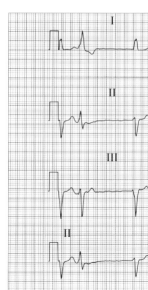

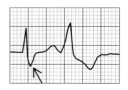

Deep wide S wave in supraventricular beat in lead V_6

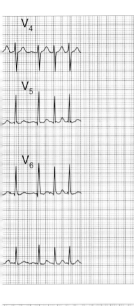

Fig. 5.1 Uncontrolled atrial fibrillation

Note
- Atrial fibrillation, with ventricular rate 153/min
- No other abnormalities
- No evidence of digoxin effect

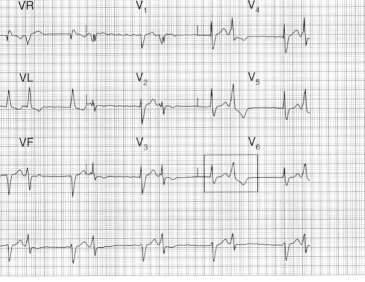

THE ECG IN DISORDERS AFFECTING THE LEFT SIDE OF THE HEART

The ECG in left atrial hypertrophy

Left atrial hypertrophy causes a double (bifid) P wave. Left atrial hypertrophy without left ventricular hypertrophy is classically due to mitral stenosis, so the bifid P wave is sometimes called 'P mitrale'. This is misleading, because most patients whose ECGs have bifid P waves either have left ventricular hypertrophy that is not obvious on the ECG or – and perhaps this is more common – have a perfectly normal heart. The bifid P wave is thus not a useful measure of left atrial hypertrophy.

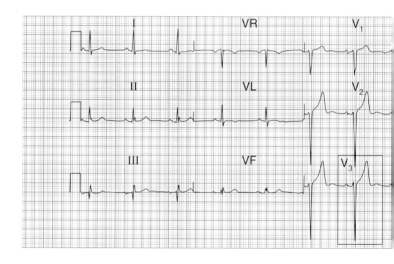

Figure 5.3 shows an ECG with a bifid P wave indicating left atrial hypertrophy. This was confirmed by echocardiography in the patient, who also had concentric left ventricular hypertrophy due to hypertension.

Significant mitral stenosis usually – but not always – leads to atrial fibrillation, so no P waves, bifid or otherwise, can be seen. Occasional patients, such as the one whose ECG is shown in Figure 5.4, develop pulmonary hypertension and remain in sinus rhythm. There is then a combination of a bifid P wave with evidence of right ventricular hypertrophy. This combination does allow a confident diagnosis of severe mitral stenosis.

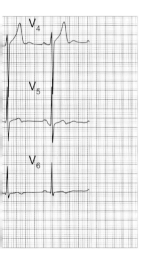

Fig. 5.3 Left atrial hypertrophy and left ventricular hypertrophy

Note
- Sinus rhythm
- Bifid P waves
- Normal axis
- Tall QRS complexes
- Inverted T waves in lead V_6, suggesting left ventricular hypertrophy

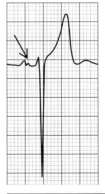

Bifid P wave in lead V_3

319

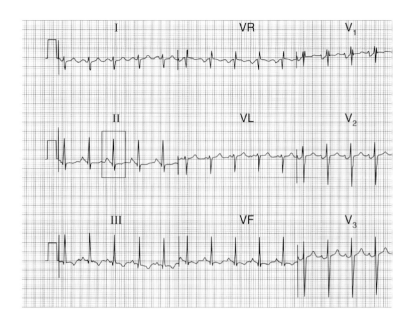

The ECG in left ventricular hypertrophy

Left ventricular hypertrophy may be caused by hypertension, aortic stenosis or incompetence, or mitral incompetence.

The ECG features of left ventricular hypertrophy are:

- An increased height of the QRS complex
- Inverted T waves in the leads that 'look at' the left ventricle: I, VL, and V_5–V_6.

Left axis deviation is not uncommon, but is due more to fibrosis causing left anterior hemiblock than to the left ventricular hypertrophy itself. The ECG is, in fact, a poor guide to the severity of left ventricular hypertrophy.

The so-called 'voltage criteria' for left ventricular hypertrophy are based on the height of the R waves and the depth of the S waves in the chest leads. Left ventricular hypertrophy is

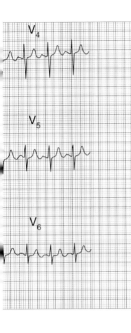

Fig. 5.4 Mitral stenosis and pulmonary hypertension

Note
- Sinus rhythm
- Bifid P wave (best seen in lead II)
- Right axis deviation
- Partial RBBB pattern
- Persistent S wave in lead V_6

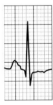

Bifid P wave in lead II

supposedly present if any R or any S wave exceeds 25 mm, or if the height of the tallest R wave plus the depth of the deepest S wave exceeds 35 mm. These criteria are essentially useless – they would frequently lead to a diagnosis of left ventricular hypertrophy in perfectly healthy young men, and even in those who are not athletic (Fig. 5.5).

The most important cause of severe left ventricular hypertrophy is aortic valve disease: when aortic stenosis or incompetence causes left ventricular hypertrophy, aortic valve replacement must be considered. Aortic valve disease is frequently associated with left bundle branch block (LBBB) (Fig. 5.6), which completely masks any evidence of left ventricular hypertrophy. The patient who is breathless, or who has chest pain or dizziness, and has signs of aortic valve disease and an ECG showing LBBB needs urgent investigation.

321

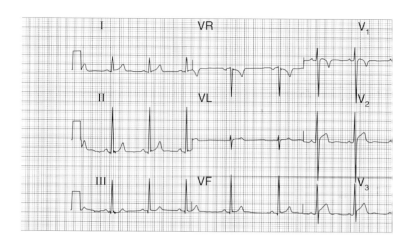

Fig. 5.6 Left bundle branch block with aortic stenosis

Note

- Sinus rhythm
- Normal axis
- Broad QRS complexes with LBBB pattern
- Very deep S waves in lead V_3
- Inverted T waves in leads I, VL, V_5, V_6

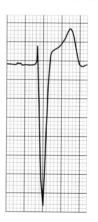

Broad QRS complex
and deep S wave in
lead V_3

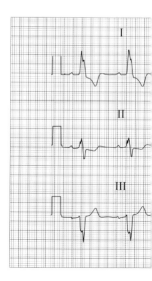

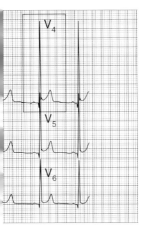

Fig. 5.5 Probably normal ECG

Note
- Sinus rhythm
- Normal axis
- Very tall R waves (meeting 'voltage criteria' for left ventricular hypertrophy)
- No other evidence of left ventricular hypertrophy

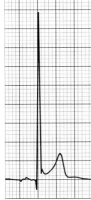

Tall R wave in lead V$_4$

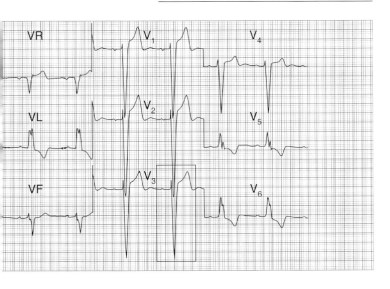

The complete ECG picture of left ventricular hypertrophy is easy to recognize. The ECG in Figure 5.7 is from a patient with severe and untreated hypertension. It shows the 'voltage criteria' which, when combined with the T wave inversion, probably are significant. In this case, the small Q waves in the lateral leads are 'septal' and do not indicate a previous infarction. Note that the T wave inversion is most prominent in lead V_6, and becomes progressively less so in leads V_5 and V_4. This pattern of T wave inversion is sometimes referred to as 'left ventricular strain', but this is an old-fashioned and essentially meaningless term.

Unfortunately the severity of ECG changes is an unreliable guide to the importance of the underlying cardiac problem. The ECG in Figure 5.8 shows lateral T wave inversion, but does not meet the 'voltage criteria', in a patient with moderate aortic stenosis (aortic valve gradient 60 mmHg).

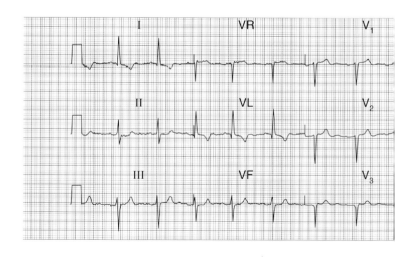

In contrast, the ECG in Figure 5.9 is from a patient with severe aortic stenosis and an aortic valve > 120 mmHg, yet it shows little to suggest severe left ventricular hypertrophy.

The main problem is differentiating lateral T wave changes due to left ventricular hypertrophy from those due to ischaemia; this has been discussed in Chapter 4. The history and physical examination become extremely important, and the ECG must not be viewed in isolation. The ECG in Figure 5.10 is from a patient with chest pain that was compatible with, but not diagnostic of, angina and who had physical signs suggesting mild aortic stenosis. The T wave inversion is more prominent in leads V_4 and V_5 than in V_6, and is present in V_3. The T waves are upright in leads I and VL. These changes point to ischaemia rather than left ventricular hypertrophy, and ischaemia proved to be present in this patient.

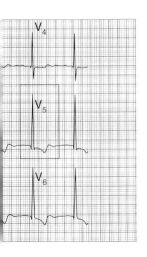

Fig. 5.7 Left ventricular hypertrophy

Note
- Sinus rhythm
- Voltage criteria for left ventricular hypertrophy
- Inverted T waves in leads I, VL, V_5, V_6

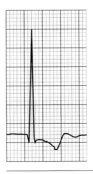

Tall R wave and inverted T wave in lead V_5

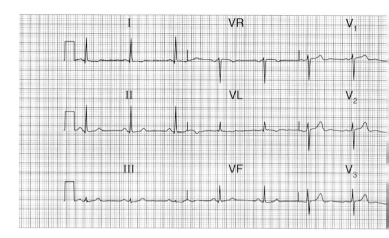

Fig. 5.9 ?Left ventricular hypertrophy with severe aortic stenosis

Note
- Sinus rhythm
- Normal axis
- Voltage criteria for left ventricular hypertrophy not met
- Minor ST segment/T wave changes in leads I, VL, V₆

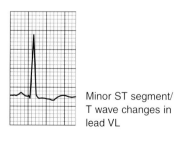

Minor ST segment/ T wave changes in lead VL

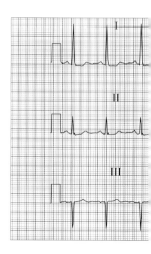

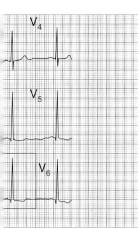

Fig. 5.8 Left ventricular hypertrophy

Note
- Sinus rhythm
- Normal axis
- Voltage criteria for left ventricular hypertrophy not met
- Inverted T waves in leads I, VL, V$_6$

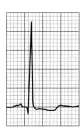

Normal R wave and inverted T wave in lead V$_6$

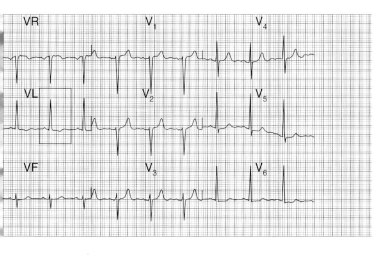

327

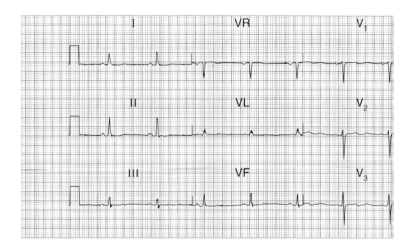

The ECG in Figure 5.11 is from a patient with hypertension and breathlessness. He was shown to have left ventricular hypertrophy and coronary disease, but all the changes here could have been due to left ventricular hypertrophy alone.

When a breathless patient has an ECG with gross lateral T wave changes (Fig. 5.12), hypertrophic cardiomyopathy is a possibility.

Lateral T wave changes associated with left anterior hemiblock often accompany left ventricular hypertrophy. However, there was no echocardiographic evidence of this in the patient whose ECG is shown in Figure 5.13. Here the changes must be due to conducting system disease.

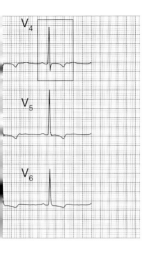

Fig. 5.10 Probable ischaemia

Note
- Sinus rhythm
- Normal axis
- T wave inversion in leads II, V_3–V_6, but most prominent in V_4, V_5

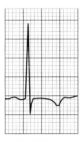

Inverted T wave in lead V_4

Another example of a conducting tissue abnormality that could be mistaken for left ventricular hypertrophy is the Wolff–Parkinson–White (WPW) syndrome. The ECG in Figure 5.14 is from a young man with WPW syndrome type B. There is left ventricular hypertrophy according to 'voltage criteria', and there is also lateral T wave inversion, but the diagnosis is made from the short PR intervals and the delta waves. The height of the QRS complexes and the T wave inversion in this situation do not indicate left ventricular hypertrophy.

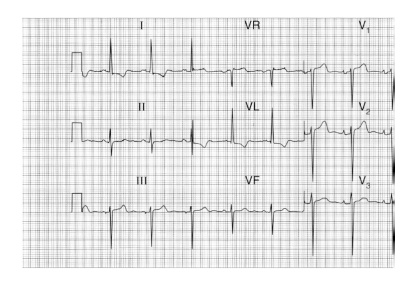

Fig. 5.12 **Hypertrophic cardiomyopathy**

Note
- Sinus rhythm
- Bifid P wave, best seen in lead V_4
- Voltage criteria for left ventricular hypertrophy not met
- Gross T wave inversion in leads V_4–V_6

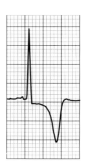

Normal R wave and dramatic T wave inversion in lead V_5

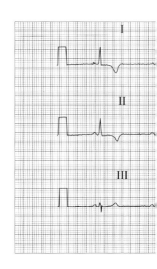

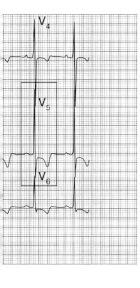

Fig. 5.11 ?Left ventricular hypertrophy, ?ischaemia

Note
- Sinus rhythm
- Bifid P waves, best seen in lead I
- Normal axis
- T wave inversion in leads I, VL, V_3–V_6, but most prominent in V_5

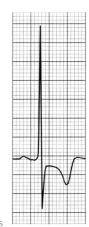

Maximal T wave inversion in lead V_5

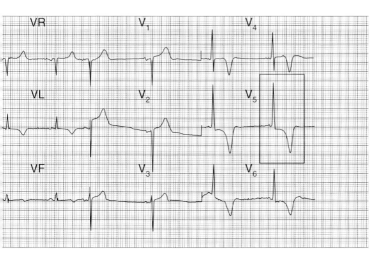

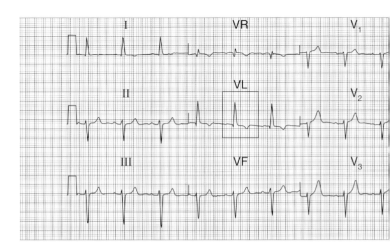

Fig. 5.14 Wolff–Parkinson–White syndrome (no left ventricular hypertrophy)

Note

- Short PR interval
- Broad QRS complexes with delta waves
- Very tall R waves
- Inverted T waves in leads I, II, VL, V_4–V_6

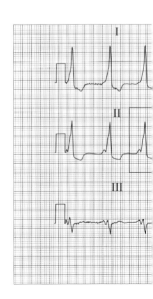

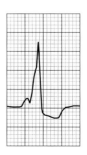

Short PR interval and delta wave in lead II

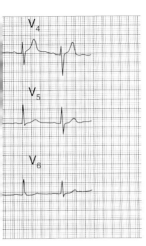

Fig. 5.13 Left anterior hemiblock

Note
- Sinus rhythm
- Left axis deviation
- Inverted T waves in leads I, VL

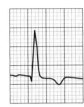

Inverted T wave in lead VL

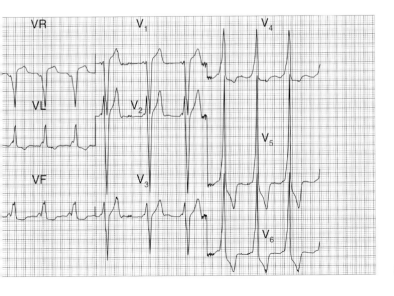

THE ECG IN DISORDERS AFFECTING THE RIGHT SIDE OF THE HEART

The ECG in right atrial hypertrophy

Right atrial hypertrophy causes tall and peaked P waves. There is, in fact, such variation within the normal range of P waves that the diagnosis of right atrial hypertrophy is difficult to make. Its presence can be inferred when peaked P waves are associated with the ECG changes of right ventricular hypertrophy. Evidence of right atrial hypertrophy without right ventricular hypertrophy will usually only be seen in patients with tricuspid stenosis (Fig. 5.15).

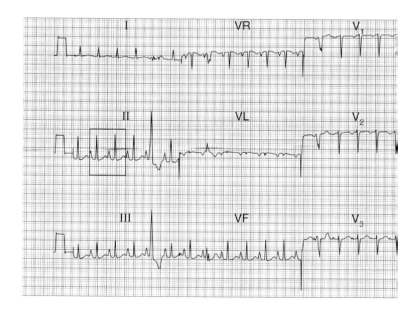

The ECG in Figure 5.16 is from a patient with right atrial and right ventricular hypertrophy due to severe chronic obstructive pulmonary disease.

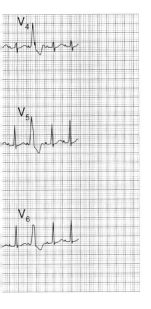

Fig. 5.15 Right atrial hypertrophy

Note
- Sinus rhythm with occasional aberrant conduction
- Tall and peaked P waves
- No other abnormality

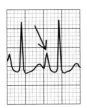

Peaked P wave in lead II

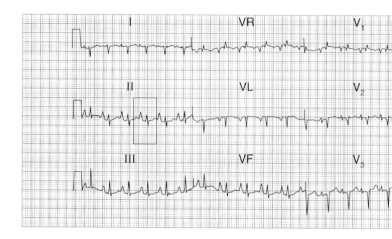

The ECG in right ventricular hypertrophy

Right ventricular hypertrophy can be the result of chronic lung disease (e.g. chronic obstructive airways disease, bronchiectasis), pulmonary embolism (especially when repeated episodes cause thromboembolic pulmonary hypertension), idiopathic pulmonary hypertension, or congenital heart disease. None of these has a specific ECG abnormality.

The ECG changes associated with right ventricular hypertrophy are:

- Right axis deviation
- A dominant R wave (i.e. the R wave height is greater than the S wave depth) in lead V_1
- 'Clockwise rotation' of the heart: as the right ventricle occupies more of the anterior surface of the chest and the septum is displaced laterally, the transition of the QRS complex in the chest leads from a right to a left ventricular configuration occurs between leads V_4 and V_6 instead of in V_2–V_4. There is thus a persistent S wave in lead V_6, which normally does not show an S wave at all. This change is called 'clockwise rotation' because, seen from the feet, the heart seems to have turned clockwise within the chest.

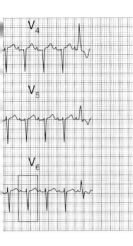

Fig. 5.16 Right atrial and right ventricular hypertrophy

Note
- Peaked P waves, especially in lead II
- Right axis deviation
- Persistent S waves in lead in V_6 (clockwise rotation) suggest chronic lung disease

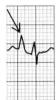

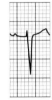

Peaked P wave in lead II

Persistent S wave in lead V_6

- Inversion of the T wave in leads that 'look at' the right ventricle: V_1, and V_2, and occasionally V_3.

In extreme cases it is easy to diagnose right ventricular hypertrophy from the ECG. The ECG in Figure 5.17 came from a patient incapacitated by breathlessness due to primary pulmonary hypertension.

As with the ECG in left ventricular hypertrophy, none of the ECG changes of right ventricular hypertrophy individually provide unequivocal evidence of right ventricular hypertrophy (see Table 5.2). Conversely, it is possible to have marked right ventricular hypertrophy without all the ECG features being present. Minor degrees of right axis deviation are seen in normal people, and a dominant R wave in lead V_1 is occasionally seen in normal people, although it is never more than 3 or 4 mm tall. A dominant R wave in lead V_1 may also indicate a 'true posterior' myocardial infarction (see Ch. 4). There may be variation in the T wave inversion in leads V_1 and V_2 in normal subjects (see Ch. 2) and, particularly in black people, the T wave can be inverted in leads V_2 and V_3.

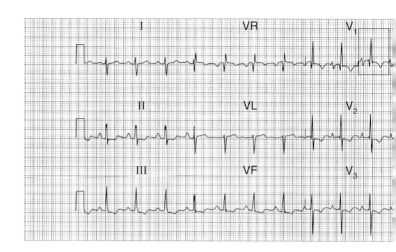

Table 5.2 Possible alternative causes of the ECG appearance of right ventricular hypertrophy

ECG feature	Cause
Right axis deviation	Normal in tall thin people
Dominant R wave in lead V$_1$	Normal variant Posterior infarction Wolff–Parkinson–White syndrome Right bundle branch block of any cause
Inverted T waves in leads V$_1$, V$_2$	Normal variant, especially in black people Anterior non-Q wave infarction Wolff–Parkinson–White syndrome Right bundle branch block of any cause
	Cardiomyopathy
Apparent clockwise rotation	Dextrocardia

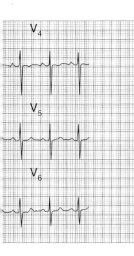

Fig. 5.17 Marked right ventricular hypertrophy

Note
- Sinus rhythm
- Peaked P waves
- Right axis deviation
- Dominant R waves in lead V_1
- Persistent S waves in lead V_6

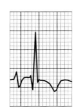

Dominant R wave in lead V_1

The ECG in Figure 5.18 shows a dominant R wave in lead V_1 but no other evidence of right ventricular hypertrophy. This could indicate a posterior myocardial infarction (see Ch. 4), but this trace was from a young man who was asymptomatic, who had no abnormalities on examination, and whose echocardiogram was normal. This is a normal variant.

The ECG in Figure 5.19 is from a young woman who had become progressively more breathless since the birth of her baby 4 months previously. She had had no chest pain. No previous ECGs were available. The anterior T wave changes could be a normal variant in a black woman. T wave inversion in leads V_3–V_4 could indicate anterior ischaemia, but the important point here is that the T wave inversion is most prominent in leads V_1 and V_2, and becomes progressively less in V_3 and V_4. This is characteristic of T wave inversion due to right ventricular hypertrophy. In this case the T wave inversion, combined with right axis deviation and a persistent S wave in lead V_6, suggests right ventricular hypertrophy. The patient was shown to have had recurrent small pulmonary emboli.

339

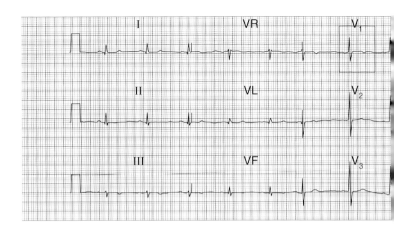

Fig. 5.19 Right ventricular hypertrophy

Note

- Sinus rhythm
- Right axis deviation
- No dominant R waves in lead V_1
- Inverted T waves in leads V_1–V_4, maximal in lead V_1
- Persistent S waves in lead V_6

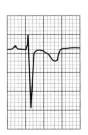

Inverted T wave in lead V_2

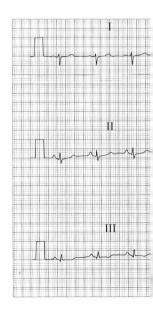

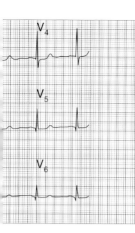

Fig. 5.18 Probable normal variant

Note
- Sinus rhythm
- Normal axis
- Dominant R waves in lead V_1
- Inverted T waves in lead III

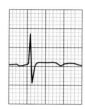

Dominant R wave in lead V_1

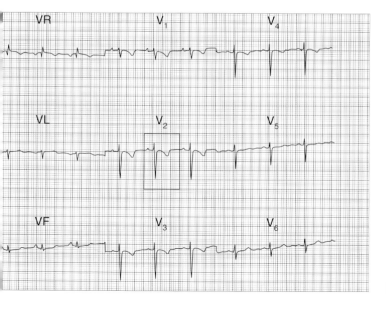

A prominent S wave in lead V_6 is sometimes called 'persistent' because this lead should show a pure left ventricular type of complex with a dominant R wave and no S wave. The 'transition point', when the R and S waves are equal, indicates the position of the interventricular septum and this is normally under the position of lead V_3 or V_4. In the ECG in Figure 5.20 a 'transition point' is not present at all, and lead V_6 shows a small R wave and a dominant S wave. This is due to the right ventricle underlying more of the precordium than usual. This change is characteristic of chronic lung disease.

When breathlessness is accompanied by a sudden change in rotation, a pulmonary embolus is likely. The ECG in Figure 5.21 is

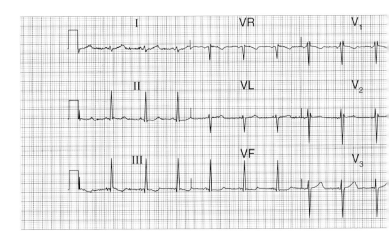

from a patient who had had a normal preoperative ECG but who developed breathlessness with atrial fibrillation a week after cholecystectomy. The deep S wave in lead V_6 is the pointer towards a pulmonary embolus being the cause of the atrial fibrillation.

As with the ECG in left ventricular hypertrophy, it is the appearance of changes in serial recordings that provides the best evidence of minor or moderate degrees of right ventricular hypertrophy. In the majority of cases in which the ECG suggests right ventricular hypertrophy, it is not possible to diagnose the underlying disease process with certainty.

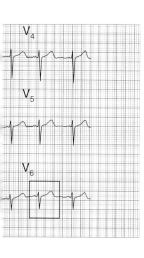

Fig. 5.20 Chronic lung disease

Note
- Sinus rhythm
- Right axis deviation
- Prominent S waves in lead V_6
- Nonspecific T wave changes in leads III and VF

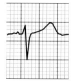

Persistent S wave in lead V_6

343

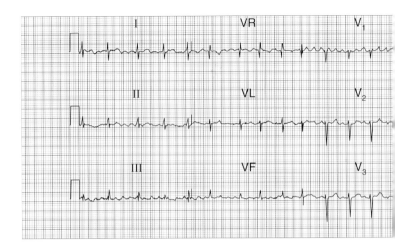

THE ECG IN CONGENITAL HEART DISEASE

The ECG provides a limited amount of help in the diagnosis of congenital heart disease by showing which chambers of the heart are enlarged. It is important to remember (see Ch. 2) that at birth the ECG of a normal infant shows a pattern of 'right ventricular hypertrophy' and this gradually disappears during the first 2 years of life.

If the infant pattern persists beyond the age of 2 years, right ventricular hypertrophy is indeed present. If there is a left ventricular, or normal adult, pattern before this age, then left ventricular hypertrophy is probably present. In older children the same criteria for left and right ventricular hypertrophy as in adults apply.

Table 5.3 lists some common congenital disorders and the associated ECG appearance.

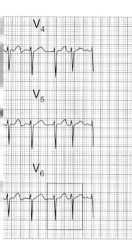

Fig. 5.21 ?Pulmonary embolus

Note
- Atrial fibrillation, ventricular rate 114/min
- Dominant S wave in lead V_6
- No other evidence of right ventricular hypertrophy

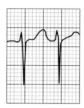

Persistent S wave in lead V_6

Table 5.3 ECG appearance in common congenital disorders

ECG appearance	Congenital disorder
Right ventricular hypertrophy	Pulmonary hypertension of any cause (e.g. Eisenmenger's syndrome) Severe pulmonary stenosis Fallot's tetralogy Transposition of the great arteries
Left ventricular hypertrophy	Aortic stenosis Coarctation of the aorta Mitral regurgitation Obstructive cardiomyopathy
Biventricular hypertrophy	Ventricular septal defect
Right atrial hypertrophy	Tricuspid stenosis
Right bundle branch block	Atrial septal defect Complex defects
Left axis deviation	Endocardial cushion defects Corrected transposition

345

The ECG in Figure 5.22 shows all the features of severe right ventricular hypertrophy: it came from a boy with severe pulmonary stenosis.

The ECG in Figure 5.23 shows left ventricular hypertrophy, and was recorded in an 8-year-old with severe aortic stenosis.

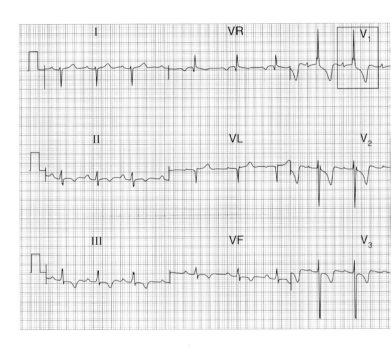

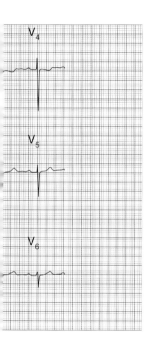

Fig. 5.22 Pulmonary stenosis

Note
- Sinus rhythm
- Right axis deviation
- Dominant R waves in lead V_1
- Persistent S waves in lead V_6
- Inverted T waves in leads V_1–V_4

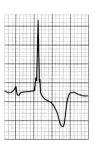

Dominant R wave in lead V_1

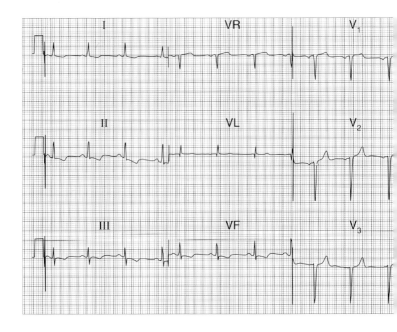

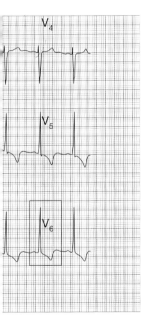

Fig. 5.23 Left ventricular hypertrophy

Note
- Sinus rhythm
- Normal axis
- Left ventricular hypertrophy according to voltage criteria
- T wave inversion in leads I, V_5–V_6

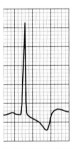

Tall R wave and inverted T wave in lead V_6

The ECG in Figure 5.24 shows right ventricular hypertrophy, and came from a young woman who had had a partial correction of Fallot's tetralogy 20 years previously.

The ECG in Figure 5.25 suggests right atrial hypertrophy and shows RBBB. It came from a teenager with Ebstein's anomaly and an atrial septal defect.

It is usually fairly obvious that a patient has congenital heart disease of some sort, but the condition that may be missed is an

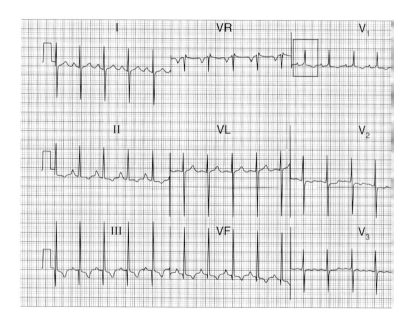

atrial septal defect. The ECG in Figure 5.26 is from a 50-year-old woman who complained of mild but increasing breathlessness. She had a rather nonspecific systolic murmur at the left sternal edge. Her GP recorded an ECG which showed RBBB, and as a result she had an echocardiogram which showed an atrial septal defect.

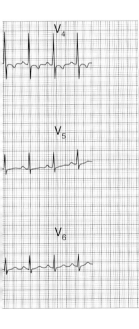

Fig. 5.24 Right ventricular hypertrophy in Fallot's tetralogy

Note
- Leads V_1–V_3 recorded at half sensitivity
- Sinus rhythm
- Right axis deviation
- Dominant R waves in lead V_1
- T wave inversion in leads II, III, VF, V_1–V_4

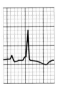

Dominant R wave in lead V_1

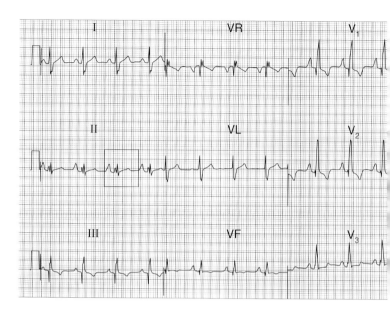

Fig. 5.26 Right bundle branch block with atrial septal defect

Note
- Sinus rhythm
- Normal axis
- QRS complex duration within normal limits (108 ms)
- RBBB pattern

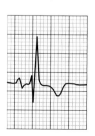

RBBB pattern in lead V$_1$

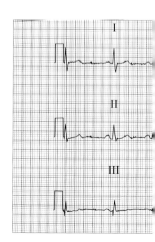

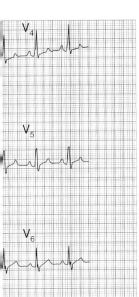

Fig. 5.25 Right atrial hypertrophy, right bundle branch block, in Ebstein's anomaly

Note
- Sinus rhythm
- Peaked P waves in lead II
- Broad QRS complexes with RBBB pattern

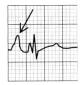

Peaked P wave in lead II

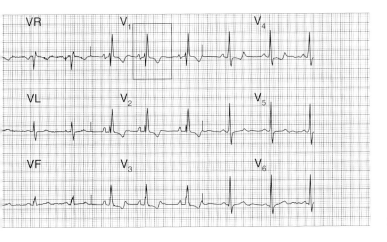

What to do

In most patients with breathlessness, the ECG does not contribute very much to diagnosis and management and the important thing is to treat the patient and not the ECG.

The ECG cannot diagnose heart failure, although heart failure is unlikely if the ECG is totally normal. By demonstrating ischaemia or enlargement of one or more of the cardiac chambers, the ECG may help to identify the underlying disease that requires treatment. However, the symptoms of acute heart failure need empirical treatment whatever the ECG shows, and this should not be delayed while an ECG is being recorded.

Similarly, while the ECG can provide confirmatory evidence that breathlessness is due to a pulmonary embolus or chronic lung disease, it is an unreliable way of making this diagnosis and treatment cannot depend on the ECG.

The ECG will not help in the diagnosis of anaemia, though it may show ischaemic changes.

In general then, the management of the breathless patient does not depend on the ECG unless breathlessness is due to heart failure which is secondary to an arrhythmia. The ECG is then essential both for diagnosis and for monitoring the response to therapy.

6

The effect of non-cardiac disease on the ECG

INTRODUCTION

The ECG is not a good method for investigating or diagnosing any condition that is not primarily cardiac. However, some generalized diseases affect the ECG – it is important to recognize this, and not assume that a patient has heart disease simply because his or her ECG seems abnormal.

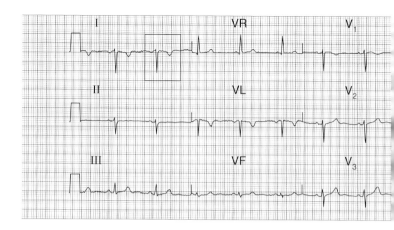

ARTEFACTS IN ECG RECORDINGS

Improper electrode placement

If the electrodes are wrongly attached to the limbs, there will be abnormalities in the ECG recorded in the limb leads, but not in the chest leads. In particular, the cardiac axis may seem bizarre.

Improper electrode attachment should be suspected and the recording repeated when the P wave is upside down in leads other than VR, despite the patient being in sinus rhythm (see Fig. 6.1). Whenever the cardiac axis is difficult to calculate, it is prudent to repeat the ECG.

Dextrocardia causes abnormalities in the limb leads similar to those caused by improper electrode attachment, but the pattern in the chest leads is also abnormal (Ch. 2).

The effects of abnormal muscle movement

The contraction of any muscle is initiated by depolarization and therefore involves electrical changes. Although ECG recorders are designed to be especially sensitive to the electrical frequencies of cardiac muscle contraction, the ECG will also record the contraction of skeletal muscles. The most common pattern of

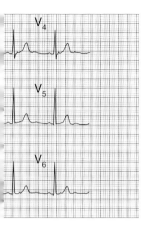

Fig. 6.1 Misplaced limb leads

Note
- Sinus rhythm
- Inverted P wave in lead I
- Axis impossible to determine
- Inverted T waves in leads I, VL
- Chest leads normal

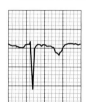

Inverted P and T waves in lead I

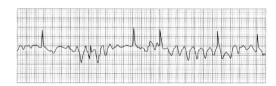

Fig. 6.2 Parkinsonism

Note
- Muscle tremor at 5/s gives an appearance resembling atrial flutter
- The irregular QRS complexes may indicate that the rhythm is actually atrial fibrillation
- This record demonstrates the importance of looking at the patient as well as the ECG

'ECG abnormality' is a high-frequency oscillation due to general muscular tension in a patient who is not properly relaxed.

Sustained involuntary tremors, such as those associated with Parkinsonism (Fig. 6.2) cause rhythmic ECG abnormalities that may be confused with cardiac arrhythmias.

357

Hypothermia

Hypothermia causes shivering, and therefore muscle artefact. However, there can be other changes in the ECG and the characteristic of hypothermia is the 'J wave'. This is a small hump seen at the end of the QRS complex.

The ECG in Figure 6.3 was recorded from a 76-year-old woman who was admitted to hospital with a temperature of 30° after lying for a prolonged period in a freezing house after a fall. She initially

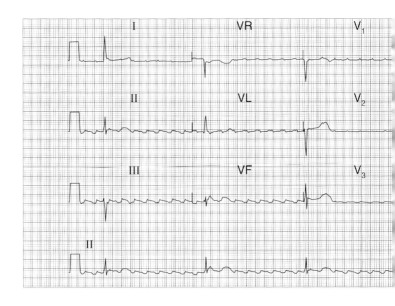

had a heart rate of 26/min and the rhythm was atrial flutter. J waves can be seen in the lateral chest leads. On re-warming she began to shiver, and despite the muscle artefact can be seen to have reverted to sinus rhythm with first degree block. J waves are still visible (Fig. 6.4). When her temperature had returned to normal, the PR interval normalized and the J waves disappeared (Fig. 6.5).

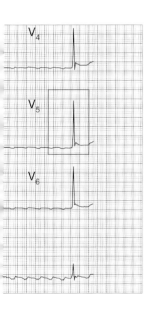

Fig. 6.3 Atrial flutter, hypothermia

Note
- Atrial flutter with ventricular rate 26/min
- J waves visible in leads V_4–V_6

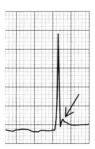

J wave in lead V_5

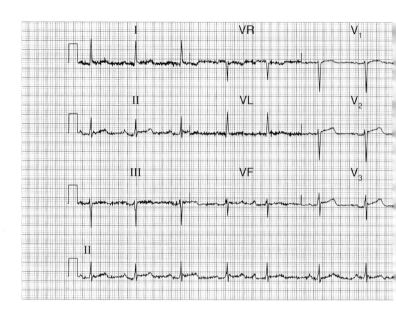

Fig. 6.5 Re-warming after hypothermia

Note

- Same patient as in Figures 6.3 and 6.4
- Patient is now in sinus rhythm with a normal PR interval.
- J waves have disappeared.
- There are some nonspecific ST segment and T wave changes in leads I, II, VL, V_6

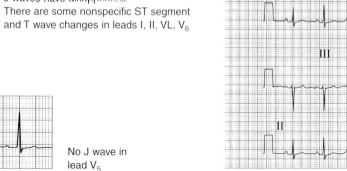

360   No J wave in lead V_5

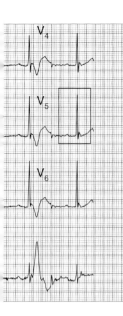

Fig. 6.4 Hypothermia

Note
- Same patient as in Figures 6.3 and 6.5
- Sinus rhythm is restored
- Patient has begun to shiver (muscle artefact in the limb leads, with a further artefact in the penultimate complex)
- First degree block
- J waves still visible

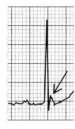

J wave in lead V_5

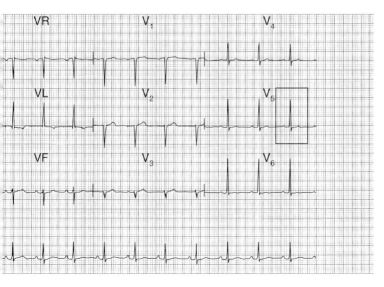

THE ECG IN SYSTEMIC DISEASES

Cardiac involvement in a generalized disorder, particularly one that causes infiltration or the deposition of abnormal substances in the myocardium, causes arrhythmias and conduction defects.

Thyroid disease

Thyrotoxicosis is probably the most common non-cardiac disorder that may present as a cardiac problem. Particularly in old age, it may cause atrial fibrillation. There is usually a rapid ventricular response which is difficult to control with digoxin (Fig. 6.6). An elderly patient may complain of palpitations or the symptoms of heart failure, and arterial embolization may occur. The usual symptoms of thyrotoxicosis may be mild or even absent.

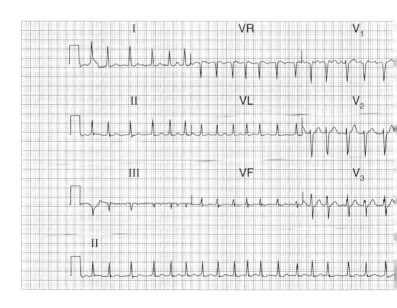

Malignancy

Metastatic deposits in and around the heart can cause virtually any arrhythmia or conduction disturbance. Malignancy is the most common cause of a large pericardial effusion, and a combination of atrial fibrillation and small complexes on the ECG suggest a malignant pericardial effusion. The ECG in Figure 6.7 is from a 60-year-old man with metastatic bronchial carcinoma.

With large effusions, the heart can rock with each beat within the effusion, causing alternate large and small QRS complexes. This is called 'electrical alternans'. The ECG in Figure 6.8 is from another patient with carcinoma of the bronchus, who presented with a supraventricular tachycardia. Electrical alternans suggests the presence of a pericardial effusion, though in this case the QRS complexes are normal size.

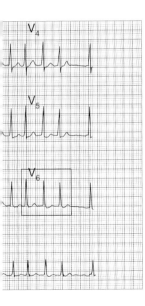

Fig. 6.6 Thyrotoxicosis

Note
- Atrial fibrillation
- Ventricular rate 153/min
- Some ST segment depression in leads V_5, V_6: ?digoxin effect
- No other abnormalities

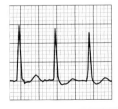

Rapid ventricular rate in lead V_6

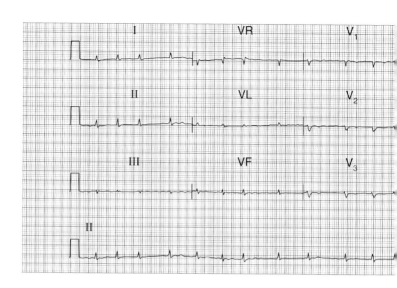

Fig. 6.8 Electrical alternans

Note

- Narrow complex tachycardia at 200/min (junctional tachycardia)
- Alternate large and small QRS complexes

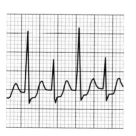

Alternate large and small QRS complexes in lead II

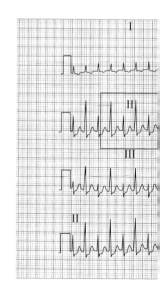

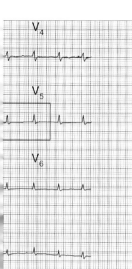

Fig. 6.7 Malignant pericardial effusion

Note
- Atrial fibrillation
- Generally small QRS complexes
- Widespread T wave flattening

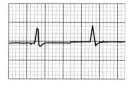

Small QRS complexes and flat T waves in lead V_5

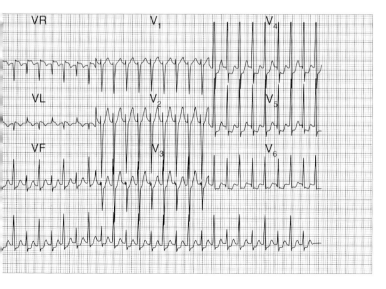

THE EFFECTS OF SERUM ELECTROLYTE ABNORMALITIES ON THE ECG

Although abnormal levels of serum potassium, magnesium and calcium can affect the ECG, the 'classical' changes are rarely seen. Occasionally an ECG may suggest that the electrolytes should be checked, but the range of normality in the ECG is so great that an ECG is an unrealistic guide to electrolyte balance. Table 6.1 summarizes the ECG changes that may occur with electrolyte imbalance.

Potassium

Hyperkalaemia may cause arrhythmias, including ventricular fibrillation or asystole; flattening of the P waves; widening of the QRS complexes; depression or loss of the ST segment; and, particularly, symmetrical peaking of the T waves. The ECG in Figure 6.9 is from a patient with renal failure and a potassium

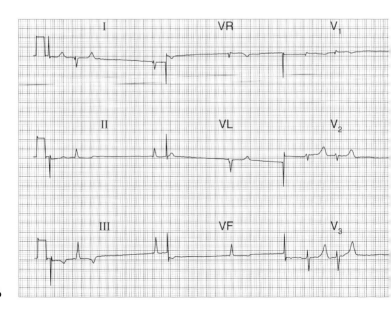

Table 6.1 The effects of electrolyte imbalance on the ECG

Electrolyte	Effect of abnormal serum electrolyte level on ECG	
	Low level	High level
Potassium or magnesium	Flat T waves Prominent U waves Depressed ST segment First or second degree block	Flat P waves Widening of QRS complexes (nonspecific intraventricular conduction delay) Tall peaked T waves Disappearance of ST segment
Calcium	Prolonged QT interval (due to long ST segment)	Short QT interval, with loss of ST segment

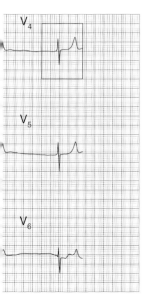

Fig. 6.9 Hyperkalaemia

Note
- No P waves
- ?Atrial fibrillation
- ?Junctional escape rhythm
- Right axis deviation
- Symmetrically peaked T waves, especially in the chest leads
- Inverted T waves in leads III, VF

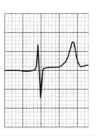

P wave absent and peaked T wave in lead V_4

367

level of 7.4 mmol. After correction of the plasma potassium level, sinus rhythm was restored and the T waves were no longer peaked (Fig. 6.10).

Remember, however, that peaked T waves are also a common finding in completely healthy patients (Fig. 6.11).

Hypokalaemia is common in patients with cardiac disease who are treated with powerful diuretics. It causes flattening of the T waves, prolongation of the QT interval, and the appearance of U waves. The ECG in Figure 6.12 was recorded from a patient with severe heart failure due to ischaemic heart disease. The serum potassium level fell to 1.9 mmol as a result of loop diuretic treatment without either potassium supplementation or the

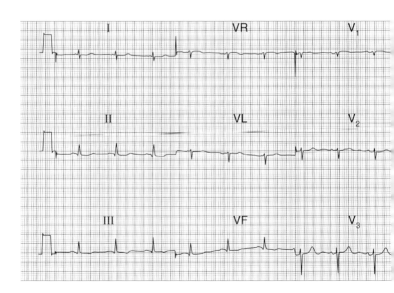

concomitant administration of an angiotensin-converting enzyme inhibitor.

Magnesium
The effects of high and low serum magnesium levels on the ECG are essentially the same as those of high and low potassium levels.

Calcium
Hypercalcaemia shortens, and hypocalcaemia prolongs, the QT interval. However, the ECG remains normal within a very wide range of serum calcium levels.

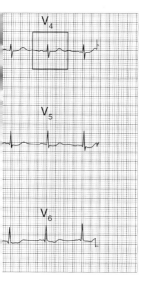

Fig. 6.10 Hyperkalaemia corrected

Note
- Same patient as in Figure 6.9
- Sinus rhythm
- ST segment depression in inferior lateral leads
- Normal T wave configuration

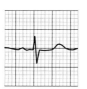

Normal P and T waves in lead V$_4$

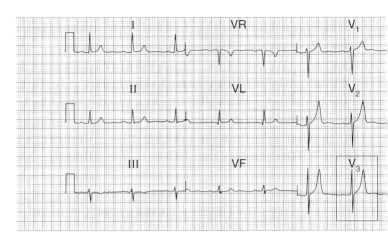

Fig. 6.12 Hypokalaemia

Note
- Leads V_1–V_6 recorded at half sensitivity
- Atrial fibrillation
- Normal axis
- Normal QRS complexes
- Flat T waves, with U waves in leads V_4, V_5

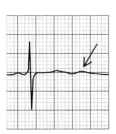

U wave in lead V_4

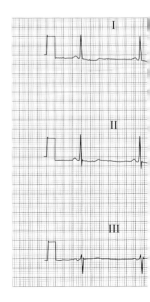

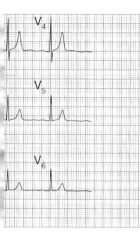

Fig. 6.11 Normal ECG

Note
- Sinus rhythm
- Normal axis
- Tall peaked T waves, resembling hyperkalaemia

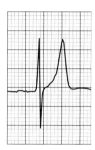

Tall, peaked T wave in lead V_3

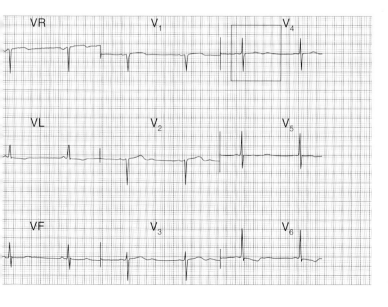

THE EFFECTS OF MEDICATION ON THE ECG

Digoxin

Atrial fibrillation is normally associated with a rapid ventricular response (sometimes inappropriately called 'fast AF'), unless conduction through the atrioventricular node is slowed by medication. Digoxin is still the best drug for controlling the ventricular rate in atrial fibrillation. The dose can be critical: the first sign of toxicity is a loss of appetite, and then the patient feels sick and vomits. Rarely, the patient complains of seeing yellow (xanthopsia). The main effect of digoxin on the ECG is downward-sloping of the ST segments, especially in the lateral leads. The appearance is sometimes referred to as a 'reverse tick' (Fig. 6.13).

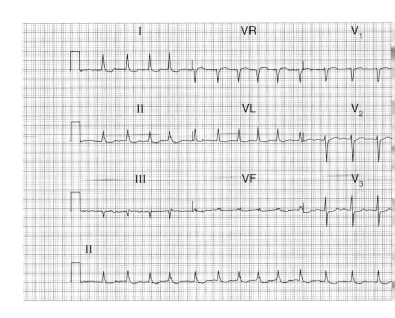

With increasing doses of digoxin the ventricular rate becomes regular and slow, and eventually complete heart block may develop. Digoxin can cause almost any arrhythmia, but especially ventricular extrasystoles and sometimes ventricular tachycardia. There is only a loose correlation between the symptoms and the ECG signs of digoxin toxicity.

The ECG in Figure 6.14 was recorded from a patient with a congestive cardiomyopathy which caused atrial fibrillation and heart failure. She was vomiting and her failure had deteriorated because her heart rate had fallen to about 40 beats/min. The ECG in Figure 6.15 shows another example of digoxin toxicity, which caused syncopal attacks due to runs of ventricular tachycardia.

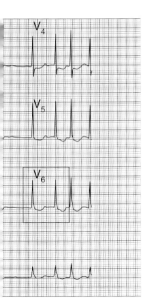

Fig. 6.13 Digoxin effect

Note
- Atrial fibrillation
- Normal axis
- Normal QRS complexes
- Downward-sloping ST segments in leads V₅, V₆

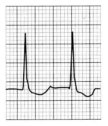

Downward-sloping ST segment in lead V₆

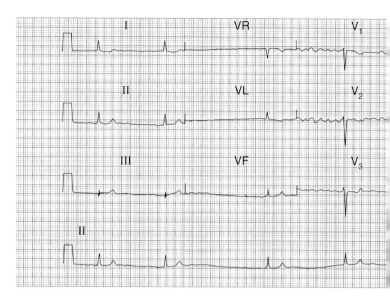

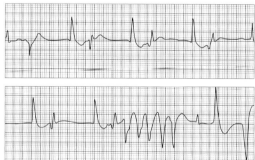

Fig. 6.15 Digoxin toxicity

Note

- The two strips form a continuous record
- Basic rhythm is atrial fibrillation: upright QRS complexes are probably the normally conducted beats
- Each upright QRS complex is followed by a predominantly downward complex, which represents a ventricular extrasystole
- In the lower strip there is a short run of ventricular tachycardia

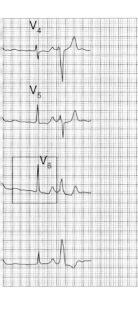

Fig. 6.14 Digoxin toxicity

Note
- Atrial fibrillation with one ventricular extrasystole
- Ventricular rate 41/min
- Normal QRS complexes
- Digoxin effect on ST segments in lead V$_6$

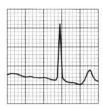

Downward-sloping ST segment in lead V$_6$

Drugs that prolong the QT interval

Over 200 drugs have been claimed to cause QT interval prolongation or torsade de pointes (TdP) ventricular tachycardia. This is particularly true of the Class I and Class III antiarrhythmic drugs. It is sensible to regard all antiarrhythmic drugs, with the exception of the beta-blockers other than sotalol, as being potentially pro-arrhythmic. While TdP ventricular tachycardia is most commonly seen in patients whose ECGs have a prolonged QT interval, in some individuals the two are apparently not related. The ECG in Figure 6.16 was recorded from a patient treated with amiodarone; the T wave changes disappeared when the drug was discontinued.

Some of the more commonly used drugs which may cause QT interval prolongation and have been associated with TdP ventricular tachycardia are:

- Antiarrhythmic drugs
  - amiodarone
  - bretylium

375

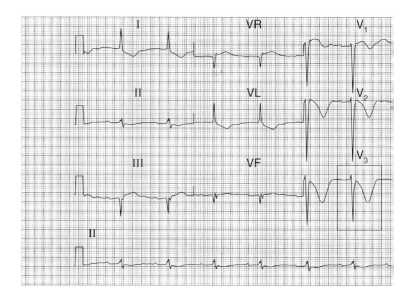

- dofetilide
- disopyramide
- flecainide
- procainamide
- propafenone
- quinidine
- sotalol
- Psychiatric drugs
  - amitryptiline
  - chlorpromazine
  - desipramine
  - haloperidol
  - imipramine
  - lithium
  - prochlorperazine
  - thioridazine
- Antimicrobial, antifungal and antimalarial drugs
  - clarithromycin

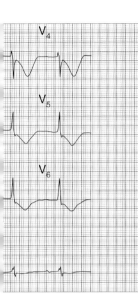

Fig. 6.16 Prolonged QT interval due to amiodarone

Note
- Sinus rhythm
- First degree block
- Normal QRS complexes
- QT interval 600 ms
- Widespread T wave inversion

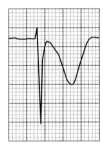

Long QT interval and inverted T wave in lead V_3

- chloroquine
- erythromycin
- ketoconazole
- quinine
- Antihistaminic drugs
  - diphenhydramine
- Others
  - alcohol
  - tacrolimus
  - tamoxifen.

Several drugs that were otherwise very useful have been withdrawn because of this problem, and the list includes the gastric pro-motility agent cisapride; the antihistamine terfenadine; the antiplatelet agent ketanserin; and the vasodilator prenylamine.

'Quinidine syncope' was recognized years before its mechanism was understood, and the ECG in Figure 6.17 is from a patient who developed TdP ventricular tachycardia while being treated with quinidine.

377

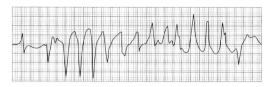

Fig. 6.17 Quinidine toxicity

Note
- A single sinus beat is followed by a run of torsade de pointes ventricular tachycardia

___

The appearance of T wave changes as, for example, in the patient needing lithium treatment whose ECG is shown in Figure 6.18, is not necessarily an indication to discontinue treatment. However, any of the drugs listed above should be discontinued if the corrected QT interval exceeds 500 ms, or if the patient has symptoms suggesting an arrhythmia. It is prudent not to use drugs known to prolong the QT interval in patients with heart disease, and combinations of QT-prolonging drugs (for example, erythromycin and ketoconazole) must definitely be avoided.

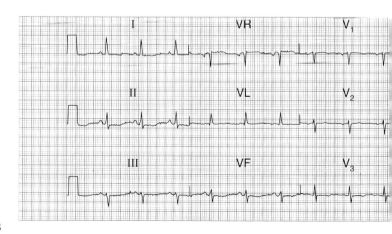

OTHER CAUSES OF AN ABNORMAL ECG

Trauma

Either penetrating (stab wound) or closed chest (usually steering wheel or seat belt) injuries can cause myocardial damage. Direct trauma to the front of the heart can lead to occlusion of the left anterior descending coronary artery, and so to the ECG of an acute anterior myocardial infarction. Seat belt injuries, however, are more usually associated with myocardial contusion, as was the case in a young woman whose ECG is shown in Figure 6.19.

Metabolic diseases

Most metabolic diseases, e.g. Addison's disease, are associated with nonspecific ST segment or T wave changes. There may be no apparent abnormality in the serum electrolytes. The ECG in Figure 6.20 is from a young girl with severe anorexia nervosa: her serum electrolytes and thyroid function were perfectly normal, but the ECG changes presumably reflect an intracellular electrolyte abnormality.

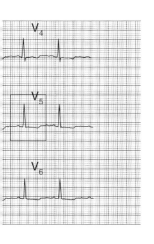

Fig. 6.18 Lithium treatment

Note
- Sinus rhythm
- Normal axis
- Normal QRS complexes
- Normal QT interval
- Widespread T wave inversion

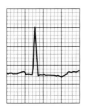

Inverted T wave in lead V_5

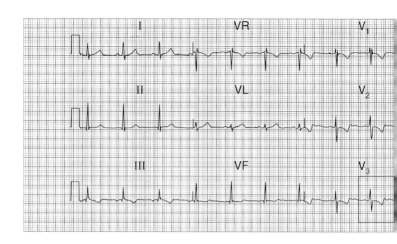

Fig. 6.20 Anorexia nervosa

Note
- Sinus rhythm at 32/min
- Artefacts in leads I, II
- Normal axis
- Normal QRS complexes
- T wave inversion and U waves in anterior chest leads

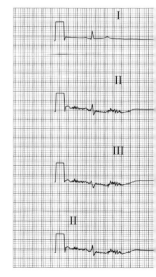

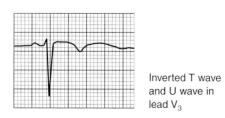

Inverted T wave and U wave in lead V₃

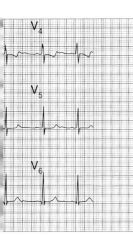

Fig. 6.19 Trauma

Note
- Sinus rhythm
- Normal axis
- Partial RBBB pattern
- Anterior T wave inversion

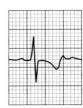

Inverted T wave in lead V₃

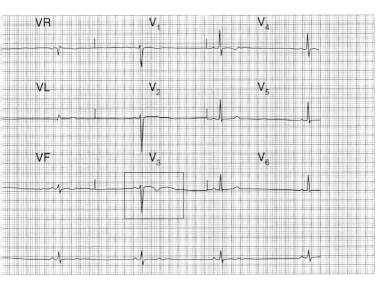

Cerebrovascular accidents

The association of a cerebrovascular accident and ECG abnormalities always suggests that the neurological problem was secondary to a cerebral embolus, which arose in the heart because of an arrhythmia or a left ventricular thrombus. However, sudden intracerebral events, particularly subarachnoid haemorrhage, can cause widespread T wave inversion. The ECG in Figure 6.21 was from a patient with subarachnoid haemorrhage.

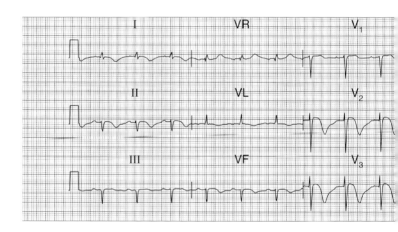

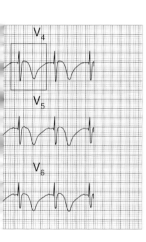

Fig. 6.21 Subarachnoid haemorrhage

Note
- Sinus rhythm
- Left axis deviation
- QT interval 600 ms
- Widespread T wave inversion

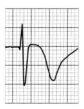

Long QT interval and inverted T wave V$_4$

Muscle disease

Many of the neuromuscular disorders are associated with a
cardiomyopathy. The ECG in Figure 6.22 is from a young man
with no cardiovascular symptoms and a clinically normal heart,
who had Friedreich's ataxia.

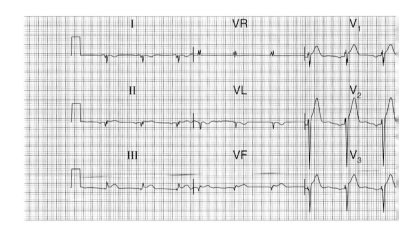

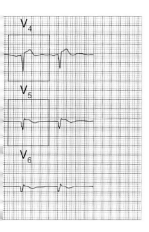

Fig. 6.22 Friedreich's ataxia

Note
- Sinus rhythm
- Right axis deviation
- Widespread T wave abnormality
- Appearances could suggest anterolateral ischaemia

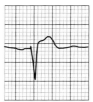 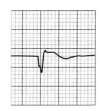

Changes in leads V₄ and V₅ suggesting an anterior infarction

385

7

Reminders

INTRODUCTION

Remember that interpreting the ECG is only a small part of making a diagnosis. The following lists are to remind you of the variations in the ECG seen in normal people, of some of the possible causes of specific ECG abnormalities, and of some of the diseases that an ECG may suggest.

WHAT CAN BE ACCEPTED AS NORMAL?

Acceptable variations in the normal ECG in adults

Rhythm
- Marked sinus arrhythmia, with escape beats
- Lack of sinus arrhythmia (normal with increasing age)
- Supraventricular extrasystoles
- Ventricular extrasystoles

P wave
- Normally inverted in lead VR
- May be inverted in lead VL

Cardiac axis
- Minor right axis deviation in tall people
- Minor left axis deviation in fat people and in pregnancy

QRS complexes in the chest leads
- Slight dominance of R wave in lead V_1, provided there is no other evidence of right ventricular hypertrophy or posterior infarction
- The R wave in the lateral chest leads may exceed 25 mm in thin fit young people
- Partial right bundle branch block (RSR^1 pattern, with QRS complexes less than 120 ms)
- Septal Q waves in leads III, VL, V_5–V_6

ST segment
- Raised in anterior leads following an S wave (high take-off ST segment)
- Depressed in pregnancy
- Nonspecific upward-sloping depression

T wave
- Inverted in lead VR and often in V_1
- Inverted in leads V_2, V_3 or even V_4 in black people
- May invert with hyperventilation
- Peaked, especially if the T waves are tall

U wave
- Normal in anterior leads when the T wave is not flattened

The ECG in normal children
At birth
- Sinus tachycardia
- Right axis deviation
- Dominant R waves in lead V_1

- Deep S waves in lead V_6
- Inverted T waves in leads V_1–V_4

At 1 year of age
- Sinus tachycardia
- Right axis deviation
- Dominant R waves in lead V_1
- Inverted T waves in leads V_1–V_2

At 2 years of age
- Normal axis
- S waves exceed R waves in lead V_1
- T waves inverted in leads V_1–V_2

At 5 years of age
- Normal QRS complexes
- T waves still inverted in leads V_1–V_2

At 10 years of age
- Adult pattern

Acceptable variations in the ECG in athletes
- Sinus arrhythmia
- 'Wandering atrial pacemaker'
- First degree block
- Wenckebach block
- Junctional rhythm
- Slight elevation of ST segments
- Tall, symmetrical T waves
- Prominent Q waves in lateral leads
- Tall R waves
- Prominent U waves

ECG in pregnancy
- Sinus tachycardia
- Supraventricular and ventricular extrasystoles
- Nonspecific ST segment/T wave changes

ASSOCIATIONS AND POSSIBLE CAUSES OF PARTICULAR ECG PATTERNS

The P wave

Absent P waves
- Atrial fibrillation
- Sinoatrial block
- Hyperkalaemia
- Junctional (AV nodal) rhythm, e.g. in sick sinus syndrome

Peaked P waves
- Lung disease
- Pulmonary embolus
- Primary pulmonary hypertension
- Pulmonary or tricuspid valve stenosis

The QRS complex

Left axis deviation
- Left anterior hemiblock
- Inferior wall infarction
- Ventricular tachycardia from left ventricular focus
- Some types of Wolff–Parkinson–White syndrome
- Congenital heart disease, e.g. endocardial cushion defects, corrected transposition

NB: Left ventricular hypertrophy in itself does not cause left axis deviation; pregnancy and obesity only cause minor degrees of left axis deviation.

Left anterior hemiblock (conduction defect in antero-superior division of left bundle branch)
Intermittent
- Any rapid supraventricular rhythm

Persistent

Fibrosis associated with:

- Ischaemic disease
- Cardiomyopathy
- Long-standing hypertension
- Long-standing congestive failure of any cause

Right axis deviation
- Right ventricular hypertrophy due to any cause
- Pulmonary embolus
- Anterolateral myocardial infarction
- Wolff–Parkinson–White syndrome with left-sided bypass
- Left posterior hemiblock (rare)

Low voltage QRS complexes
- Incorrect standardization
- Emphysema
- Obesity
- Pericardial effusion
- Myxoedema
- Hypopituitarism

Wide QRS complexes
- Rhythms with a ventricular origin (extrasystoles, tachycardias, accelerated idioventricular rhythms, escape rhythms such as complete block)
- Left anterior hemiblock
- Right bundle branch block
- Left bundle branch block

Right bundle branch block
- Seen in normal subjects
- Atrial septal defect
- Pulmonary embolus
- Cor pulmonale

Left bundle branch block
- Occasionally seen in healthy subjects
- Ischaemic heart disease
- Cardiomyopathy
- Hypertension
- Idiopathic fibrosis

Q waves
- Normal if less than 40 ms duration or 2 mm deep
- 'Septal' Q waves normal in the lateral leads
- Common in normal records in leads III, V_5–V_6
- Myocardial infarction of more than a few hours' duration

Dominant R waves in lead V_1
- Minor R wave dominance can be normal
- Associated with right bundle branch block
- Pulmonary embolus
- Right ventricular hypertrophy due to any cause
- Posterior myocardial infarction
- Myocarditis
- Wolff–Parkinson–White syndrome with left-sided pathway

The QT interval and ST segment

Long QT interval
- QT interval lengthens somewhat during sleep
- Congenital:
  - Jervell–Lange–Nielsen syndrome (includes deafness)
  - Romano–Ward syndrome (no deafness)
- Acute myocarditis due to any cause
- Acute myocardial infarction
- Cerebral injury
- Hypothermia
- Complete AV block
- Low serum calcium, potassium, or magnesium level
  Class Ia antiarrhythmic drugs, e.g. quinidine, procainamide
- Other drugs, including tricyclic antidepressants and chloroquine

Short QT interval
- Digoxin
- Hypercalcaemia
- Hyperthermia

NB: The faster the heart rate, the shorter the QT interval.

ST segment depression
- Normal if upward-sloping
- Nonspecific if concave upwards and the depression is < 2 mm
- Digoxin if downward-sloping
- Ischaemic if horizontal

ST segment elevation
- Normal variant (high take-off ST segment)
- Acute myocardial infarction
- Prinzmetal's angina
- Pericarditis
- Left ventricular aneurysm
- During stress testing, may be due to impaired left ventricular function

The T wave

Anterior T wave inversion

In leads V_1–V_3 or V_4
- Normal in black people and children
- Right bundle branch block
- Pulmonary embolism

In leads V_2–V_5
- Non-Q wave myocardial infarction
- Hypertrophic cardiomyopathy
- Subarachnoid haemorrhage
- Lithium treatment

In leads V_4–V_6
- Left ventricular hypertrophy
- Ischaemia
- Associated with left bundle branch block

Lateral T wave inversion
- Ischaemia
- Left ventricular hypertrophy
- Associated with left bundle branch block

Flattening of the T wave
- Pericardial effusion
- Hypokalaemia
- Hypothyroidism

The U wave
- May be normal
- Hypokalaemia
- Hypocalcaemia
- Hypothyroidism

Tachycardias and bradycardias

Slow rhythms
- Sinus bradycardia
- Sick sinus syndrome
- Second or third degree block
- Escape rhythms
- Drugs

Narrow complex tachycardias
The effect of carotid sinus pressure is shown in parentheses:

- Sinus (slows)
- Atrial (arrhythmia abolished or no effect)
- Atrioventricular re-entry (junctional) (arrhythmia abolished or no effect)
- Atrial flutter (increased AV block)
- Atrial fibrillation (no effect)

Broad complex tachycardias
- Supraventricular rhythm with bundle branch block
- Ventricular tachycardia
- Accelerated idioventricular rhythm (rate < 120/min)
- Torsades de pointes ventricular tachycardia
- Wolff–Parkinson–White syndrome

Broad complex tachycardias are usually ventricular in the context of acute myocardial infarction.

Differentiation of broad complex tachycardias

Comparison with record taken in sinus rhythm
- Identification of P waves (independent P waves in ventricular tachycardia)
- QRS complex width: if > 160 ms, usually ventricular
- QRS complex regularity: if very irregular, probably atrial fibrillation with conduction defect
- Cardiac axis: left axis deviation, especially with right bundle branch block, is usually ventricular
- Any axis change compared with sinus rhythm probably indicates ventricular origin

Concordance
Ventricular tachycardia is likely if:

- the QRS complex is predominantly upward, or predominantly downward, in all the chest leads

With right bundle branch block pattern
Ventricular origin is likely in the case of:

- Left axis deviation
- Tall R waves in lead V_1
- R wave taller than R^1 in lead V_1

With left bundle branch block pattern
Ventricular origin is likely in the case of:

- QS wave (i.e. no R wave) in lead V_6

Capture beats
Narrow complex following short R–R interval (i.e. an early narrow beat interrupting a broad complex tachycardia) suggests that basic rhythm is ventricular.

Fusion beats
An intermediate QRS complex pattern arises when the ventricles are activated simultaneously by a supraventricular and a ventricular impulse.

Sick sinus syndrome variants

- Inappropriate sinus bradycardia
- Sinoatrial arrest
- Sinus node exit block
- 'Silent atrium' – junctional escape
- Bradycardia–tachycardia syndrome
- Atrial fibrillation with slow ventricular response

The ECG and the peripheral pulse

Rhythms that may underlie an apparently normal or slightly slow pulse rate
- Sinus bradycardia
- Atrial flutter with 3:1 or 4:1 block
- Second degree (2:1) block
- Complete AV block with a ventricular escape rate of about 50/min
- Sick sinus syndrome with idionodal rhythm
- Idioventricular rhythm

Rhythms that may underlie an irregular pulse
- Marked sinus arrhythmia
- Supraventricular or ventricular extrasystoles
- Atrial fibrillation
- Flutter with variable block
- Varying sinus rhythm and AV block

ECG PATTERNS WHICH MAY BE ASSOCIATED WITH SPECIFIC CONDITIONS

Congenital heart disease

Pulmonary stenosis
- Right atrial and right ventricular hypertrophy

Fallot's tetralogy
- Right atrial and right ventricular hypertrophy

395

Atrial septal defect
- Left atrial or right atrial hypertrophy
- Partial or complete right bundle branch block

Ventricular septal defect
- Normal
- Left ventricular hypertrophy

Eisenmenger's syndrome
- Right ventricular hypertrophy

Valve disease
Mitral stenosis
- Atrial fibrillation
- Left atrial hypertrophy, if in sinus rhythm
- Right ventricular hypertrophy

Mitral regurgitation
- Atrial fibrillation
- Left atrial hypertrophy, if in sinus rhythm
- Left ventricular hypertrophy

Aortic stenosis
- Left ventricular hypertrophy
- Incomplete left bundle branch block (i.e. loss of Q waves in leads V_5–V_6)
- Left bundle branch block

Aortic regurgitation
- Left ventricular hypertrophy
- Prominent but narrow Q wave in lead V_6
- Left anterior hemiblock
- Occasionally, left bundle branch block

Mitral valve prolapse
- Sinus rhythm, or wide variety of arrhythmias
- Inverted T waves in leads II, III, VF
- T wave inversion in precordial leads

- ST segment depression
- Exercise-induced ventricular arrhythmias

   NB: Abnormalities can vary in different records from the same individual.

Biventricular hypertrophy
- Left ventricular hypertrophy plus right axis deviation
- Left ventricular hypertrophy plus clockwise rotation
- Left ventricular hypertrophy with tall R waves in lead V_1

Congestive cardiomyopathy
- Arrhythmias, especially atrial fibrillation and ventricular tachycardia
- First degree block
- Right or left atrial enlargement
- Low amplitude QRS complexes
- Left anterior hemiblock
- Left bundle branch block
- Right bundle branch block
- Left ventricular hypertrophy
- Nonspecific ST segment and T wave changes

Hypertrophic cardiomyopathy
- Short PR interval
- Various rhythm disturbances, including ventricular tachycardia, ventricular fibrillation
- Left atrial hypertrophy
- Left anterior hemiblock or left bundle branch block
- Left ventricular hypertrophy
- Prolonged QT interval
- Deep T wave inversion anteriorly

Myocarditis
- Sinus tachycardias and other arrhythmias
- First, second or third degree block
- Widened QRS complexes
- Irregularity of QRS waveform
- Q waves

- Prolonged QT interval
- ST segment elevation or depression
- T wave inversion in any lead

Acute rheumatic fever
- Sinus tachycardia
- First degree block
- ST segment/T wave changes of acute myocarditis
- Changes associated with pericarditis

Pulmonary embolism
- Sinus tachycardia
- Atrial arrhythmias
- Right atrial hypertrophy
- Right ventricular hypertrophy
- Right axis deviation
- Clockwise rotation with persistent S wave in lead V_6
- Right bundle branch block
- Combination of S wave in lead I with Q wave and inverted T wave in lead III

Chronic obstructive pulmonary disease
- Small complexes
- Right atrial hypertrophy (P pulmonale)
- Right axis deviation
- Right ventricular hypertrophy
- Clockwise rotation (deep S waves in lead V_6)
- Right bundle branch block

Electrolytes

Potassium and magnesium imbalance

Low level
- Flattened T waves
- U waves
- First or second degree block
- Depressed ST segments

High level
- Flat or absent P waves
- Widening of QRS complexes
- Intraventricular conduction delay
- Tall, wide, peaked, symmetrical T waves
- Disappearance of ST segment
- Arrhythmias

Calcium imbalance

Low level
- Prolonged QT interval, due to prolonged ST segment

High level
- Short QT interval, with absent ST segment

Digoxin
- Downward-sloping ST segments
- Flattened or inverted T waves
- Short QT interval
- Almost any abnormal cardiac rhythm, but especially:
  - Sinus bradycardia
  - Paroxysmal atrial tachycardia with AV block
  - Ventricular extrasystoles
  - Ventricular tachycardia
  - Any degree of AV block

Regularization of QRS complexes in atrial fibrillation suggests toxicity.

Wolff–Parkinson–White syndrome
- Short PR interval
- Slight widening of QRS complexes: delta wave with normal terminal segment
- ST segment/T wave changes
- Arrhythmias (narrow or wide complex)
- Arrhythmia with wide, irregular complex suggests WPW syndrome with atrial fibrillation
- Right-sided pathway: sometimes, anterior T wave inversion
- Left-sided pathway: dominant R waves in leads V_1–V_6

399

Exercise testing

Stress testing may reveal:

- Patient's attitude to exercise
- Reason for exercise intolerance (breathlessness etc.)
- Ventricular performance: heart rate and blood pressure response
- Ischaemia
- Exercise-induced arrhythmias

  The ECG recorded during exercise testing is unreliable in cases of:

- Bundle branch block
- Ventricular hypertrophy
- Wolff–Parkinson–White syndrome
- Digoxin therapy
- Beta-blocker therapy

POSSIBLE CAUSES OF ECG ABNORMALITIES

Remember that there are several clinical causes of all ECG abnormalities: there is always a differential diagnosis.

Sinus tachycardia

- Pain, fright, exercise
- Hypovolaemia
- Myocardial infarction
- Heart failure
- Pulmonary embolism
- Obesity
- Lack of physical fitness
- Pregnancy
- Thyrotoxicosis
- Anaemia
- Beri-beri
- CO_2 retention
- Autonomic neuropathy
- Drugs:
  - Sympathomimetics
  - Salbutamol (including by inhalation)

- Caffeine
- Atropine

Sinus bradycardia
- Physical fitness
- Vasovagal attacks
- Sick sinus syndrome
- Acute myocardial infarction, especially inferior
- Hypothyroidism
- Hypothermia
- Obstructive jaundice
- Raised intracranial pressure
- Drugs:
  - Beta-blockers (including eye drops for glaucoma)
  - Verapamil
  - Digoxin

Sick sinus syndrome

Familial
- Isolated
- With atrioventricular conduction disturbance
- With QT interval prolongation
- Congenital

Acquired
- Idiopathic
- Coronary disease
- Rheumatic disease
- Cardiomyopathy
- Neuromuscular disease:
  - Friedreich's ataxia
  - Peroneal muscular atrophy
  - Charcot–Marie–Tooth disease
- Infiltration:
  - Amyloidosis
  - Haemochromatosis
- Collagen diseases:
  - Rheumatoid
  - Scleroderma
  - SLE

401

- Myocarditis:
  - Viral
  - Diphtheria
- Drugs:
  - Lithium
  - Aerosol propellants

Atrial fibrillation (paroxysmal or persistent)
- Rheumatic heart disease
- Thyrotoxicosis
- Alcoholism
- Cardiomyopathy
- Acute myocardial infarction
- Chronic ischaemic heart disease
- Hypertension
- Myocarditis
- Pericarditis
- Pulmonary embolism
- Pneumonia
- Cardiac surgery
- Wolff–Parkinson–White syndrome
- 'Lone'

Ventricular tachycardia
- Acute myocardial infarction
- Chronic ischaemia
- Cardiomyopathy:
  - Hypertrophic
  - Dilated
- Mitral valve prolapse
- Myocarditis
- Electrolyte imbalance
- Congenital long QT syndrome
- Drugs:
  - Antiarrhythmic
  - Digoxin
- Idiopathic

Torsade de pointes ventricular tachycardia
- Class I antiarrhythmic drugs
- Amiodarone
- Sotalol
- Tricyclic antidepressants
- And many others

Electromechanical dissociation (EMD arrest)
- Tamponade
- Drug overdose
- Electrolyte imbalance
- Hypothermia
- Pulmonary embolism
- Tension pneumothorax

Heart block
First and second degree
- Normal variant
- Increased vagal tone
- Athletes
- Sick sinus syndrome
- Acute carditis
- Ischaemic disease
- Hypokalaemia
- Lyme disease (*Borrelia burgdorferi*)
- Digoxin
- Beta-blockers
- Calcium-channel blockers

Complete block
- Idiopathic (conduction tissue fibrosis)
- Congenital
- Ischaemic disease
- Associated with aortic valve calcification
- Cardiac surgery and trauma
- Digoxin intoxication
- Bundle interruption by tumours, parasites, abscesses, granulomas, injury

Pericarditis
- Viral
- Bacterial (including tuberculosis)
- Dressler's syndrome after myocardial infarction
- Malignancy
- Uraemia
- Acute rheumatic fever
- Myxoedema
- Connective tissue diseases
- Radiotherapy

Myocarditis

Viral
- Coxsackievirus B3
- Hepatitis
- Mumps
- Influenza

Bacterial
- Septicaemia
- Tuberculosis

Rickettsial
- Scrub typhus

Mycotic
- Histoplasmosis
- Actinomycosis

Parasitic
- Chagas' disease

Prolapsing mitral valve syndrome
- Primary degeneration of chordae
- Coronary disease and papillary muscle dysfunction
- Acute carditis
- Marfan's syndrome
- Hypertrophic cardiomyopathy

- Wolff–Parkinson–White syndrome
- Hereditary long QT syndromes

Hypokalaemia
- Diuretic therapy
- Antidiuretic hormone secretion

Hyperkalaemia
- Renal failure
- Potassium-retaining diuretics (amiloride, spironolactone, triamterine)
- Angiotensin-converting enzyme inhibitors
- Liquorice
- Bartter's syndrome

Hypocalcaemia
- Hypoparathyroidism
- Severe diarrhoea
- Enteric fistulae
- Alkalosis
- Vitamin D deficiency

Hypercalcaemia
- Hyperparathyroidism
- Renal failure
- Sarcoidosis
- Malignancy
- Myeloma
- Excess vitamin D
- Thiazide diuretics

8
Conclusions

The ECG is basically easy to understand, and most of its abnormalities are perfectly logical. As in everything in biology and medicine, there are quite marked variations – in both the ECGs of normal subjects and the ECG patterns that accompany specific diseases – and it is these variations that sometimes make ECG interpretation seem difficult. These variations will be recognized with practice and as a learning mechanism there is no substitute for reporting large numbers of ECGs, whether these be normal or abnormal.

However, the key to the ECG is to use it as an adjunct to the patient's history and physical examination. When in doubt, it is better to depend on these than on the ECG and it is always the patient who should be treated, not the ECG.

Remember that most ECG abnormalities have several causes: an ECG, like a clinical problem, always has a differential diagnosis.

Now test yourself: *150 ECG problems*, a companion to this volume, gives 150 clinical scenarios with full ECGs and poses questions about ECG interpretation and patient management.

Index

Note: Page numbers in *italics* refer to figures and tables on those pages.